Cosmetic Photodynamic Therapy

Aesthetic Dermatology

Vol. 3

Series Editor

David J. Goldberg New York, N.Y.

Cosmetic Photodynamic Therapy

Volume Editor

Michael H. Gold Nashville, Tenn.

34 figures, 26 in color, and 10 tables, 2016

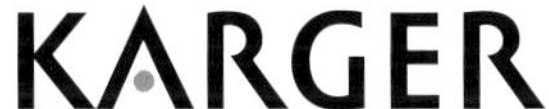

Basel · Freiburg · Paris · London · New York · Chennai · New Delhi ·
Bangkok · Beijing · Shanghai · Tokyo · Kuala Lumpur · Singapore · Sydney

Michael H. Gold, MD
Medical Director
Gold Skin Care Center
Tennessee Clinical Research Center
Nashville, Tenn., USA

Library of Congress Cataloging-in-Publication Data

Names: Gold, Michael H., editor.
Title: Cosmetic photodynamic therapy / volume editor, Michael H. Gold.
Other titles: Aesthetic dermatology (Series) ; v. 3. 2235-8609
Description: Basel ; New York : Karger, 2016. | Series: Aesthetic dermatology, ISSN 2235-8609 ; vol. 3 | Includes bibliographical references and indexes.
Identifiers: LCCN 2015045339| ISBN 9783318025569 (hard cover : alk. paper) | ISBN 9783318025576 (e-ISBN)
Subjects: | MESH: Photochemotherapy--methods. | Cosmetic Techniques. | Precancerous Conditions--drug therapy. | Skin Diseases--drug therapy.
Classification: LCC RD119 | NLM WB 480 | DDC 617.9/52--dc23 LC record available at http://lccn.loc.gov/2015045339

Bibliographic Indices. This publication is listed in bibliographic services, including Current Contents®.

www.karger.com
Printed in Germany on acid-free and non-aging paper (ISO 9706) by Kraft Druck GmbH, Ettlingen
ISSN 2235–8609
e-ISSN 2235–8595
ISBN 978–3–318–02556–9
e-ISBN 978–3–318–02557–6

Contents

VII **Preface**
Gold, M.H. (Nashville, Tenn.)

1 **A Historical Look at Photodynamic Therapy**
Gold, M.H. (Nashville, Tenn.)

8 **Photodynamic Therapy in Treating Actinic Keratosis and Photorejuvenation**
Peterson, J.D. (Katy, Tex.); Goldman, M.P. (San Diego, Calif.)

36 **Topical Methyl Aminolevulinate-Photodynamic Therapy for the Treatment of Actinic Keratoses and Photorejuvenation**
Foley, P. (Fitzroy, Vic./Carlton, Vic.)

64 **Photodynamic Therapy – Novel Cosmetic Approaches**
Munavalli, G.S. (Charlotte, N.C./Winston-Salem, N.C.); Clementoni, M.T. (Milan); Roscher, M.B. (Durban)

85 **Photodynamic Therapy for Acne Vulgaris and Sebaceous Gland Hyperplasia**
Taub, A.F. (Lincolnshire, Ill./Chicago, Ill.); Schieber, A.C. (Lincolnshire, Ill.)

103 **Chemoprevention Using Photodynamic Therapy with Aminolevulinic Acid**
Martin, G. (Kihei, Hawaii)

123 **How I Use Photodynamic Therapy with 5-Aminolevulinic Acid in My Clinical Practice**
Gilbert, D.J. (Newport Beach, Calif.)

133 **Author Index**

134 **Subject Index**

Preface

Photodynamic therapy (PDT) has become a very acceptable and useful therapy for dermatologists and others all around the world. New and exciting ways to utilize PDT continue to emerge and the future for PDT looks brighter and brighter. What began as two pathways for PDT use in dermatology, with the United States working predominantly with aminolevulinic acid (ALA) as the photosensitizer and with blue light and lasers, while the European model has been a study in the use of methyl ester of ALA with red light. The paths have now converged as far as light sources are concerned, and people have begun using the light sources interchangeably to fit the patient's needs and the circumstances of the treatment. This latest textbook on PDT brings together some of the greatest minds in the field and in the study of PDT, from all corners of the globe. PDT is truly global, and I hope that with this volume, one learns that there are wonderful therapeutic options that exist now when we use PDT, and the cosmetic outcomes, which are achieved with its use, continue to elevate PDT in every practitioner's therapeutic and cosmetic armamentarium.

As I have noted in other textbooks that I have had the privilege to edit, I am truly one of the fortunate dermatologists who has surpassed every dream and inspiration that I ever had when I began my career over 25 years ago. I want to thank Northwestern University for allowing me to be a dermatology resident under the leadership of Dr. Henry Roenigk. He pushed and guided us to be the best we can be and he, along with Drs. William Caro, June Robinson, Jerome Garden, and our beloved Ruth Frankel, inspired us and commanded us to work hard, be compassionate, and strive to give the best patient care. My fellow residents, who made me who I am, also are some of my best friends today. Thanks go to Drs. Amy Taub, Morgan Magid, David Piscasia, Dan Kaufman, Andrew Lazar, Richard Rubenstein, Neil Goldberg, and Kevin Pinski. These incredible practitioners, friends, and colleagues have been with me then and now, and I cannot thank them enough for their friendship, their encouragement, and their drive to make me a better dermatologist.

In one's career, one is fortunate to meet and work with a few really special people. I am extremely fortunate to have worked with some of the most talented and incredible dermatologists that, again, have shaped my career and have made me a better person and a better dermatologist. Thanks go to Drs. David Goldberg, Mitch Goldman, Mark Nestor, and George Martin. When it comes to PDT and what little I have contributed to the field, I must remember the late Dr. Geoffrey Shulman, the one who first sparked my interest in the field, as well as Dr. Stuart Marcus and Paul Sowyrda. Each one of these people has been a key part in my growth with PDT and dermatology.

One cannot end without thanking those who really deserve the credit for allowing me to be who I am and to do what I do. My wife Cindee, and my children Ilissa and Benjamin, along with my golden doodles Shana and Boychik, have let me be me, have let me go to places I have never dreamt I would visit, and allow me to be the best I can be. I love them all very much. And to my parents, Jerry and Anne, I am grateful for all of your teachings and guidance over my lifetime, and to have incredible parents like you.

Michael H. Gold, Nashville, Tenn.

Gold MH (ed): Cosmetic Photodynamic Therapy. Aesthet Dermatol. Basel, Karger, 2016, vol 3, pp 1–7
DOI: 10.1159/000439327

A Historical Look at Photodynamic Therapy

Michael H. Gold

Gold Skin Care Center, Tennessee Clinical Research Center, and Division of Dermatology, Department of Medicine, Vanderbilt University School of Nursing, and School of Medicine, Meharry Medical College, Nashville, Tenn., USA

Abstract

Many dermatologists who utilize photodynamic therapy (PDT) in their everyday clinical practices assume that PDT is a fairly new therapeutic modality. In fact, and surprising to many, PDT has been available in medicine since the beginning of the 20th century. In this review, we will trace some of the major roots of PDT and how it ended up in the capable hands of dermatologists, many of whom utilize the treatment on a daily basis for the well-being of their patients with a variety of skin concerns.

The beginnings of photodynamic therapy (PDT) history can be traced to the year 1900, when Raab [1] first described an experiment that was conducted with cells from *Paramecium caudatum*. He noted that the paramecium cells were not affected in any way when they were exposed to either acridine orange or a light source alone. But he noted that if the paramecium cells were exposed to the acridine orange and the light source at the same time, the same cells died within 2 h of this exposure. This was the first report of how PDT would come to be – the use of a photosensitizer, in this case acridine orange, and a light source to cause an effect on a cell, in this case, cell death.

Several years later, in 1904, von Tappeiner and Jodblauer [2] termed the expression *photodynamic effect* as they described their experiments in which an oxygen-consuming reaction in protozoa was noted after aniline dyes were applied to the protozoa with fluorescence. The following year, in 1905, Jesionek and von Tappeiner [3] reported on their experiences with a topical 5% eosin as a photosensitizer in their experiments on PDT. Topical 5% eosin was used successfully as a photosensitizer with an artificial light source to successfully treat a variety of dermatologic skin conditions common in the day, including nonmelanoma skin cancers, lupus vulgaris, and condylomata lata. The researchers postulated that the topical eosin that was being applied to the lesions could be incorporated into the cells, as was noted with acridine orange earlier, and, once in the appropriate cells, could produce a cytotoxic reaction when the lesions were exposed to an appropriate light source in the presence of oxygen. These early, pioneering experiments and studies were in fact the first reports of PDT in human subjects and became the prototype for all the future interest and scientific awareness in the field of PDT, and we are fortunate to note that dermatologic skin concerns were where the origins of the study of PDT began, which now reaches far and wide. The concept described in 1905 on which PDT works still holds steadfast today. An appropriate photosensitizer applied to the skin can be absorbed into appropriate and specific cells within the skin, and in the presence of oxygen and an appropriate light source can produce a phototoxic reaction within those skin cells, leading to a photodynamic effect and cell death in that particular cell.

Soon after these reports on what we now know was PDT, other researchers began looking at PDT and, specifically, the photosensitizers that could be used to potentially make the process even better than what had earlier been described. The PDT field turned its attention to the use of porphyrins as photosensitizers. In 1911, Hausman et al. [4] reported on the use of hematoporphyrin as a possible photosensitizer. The group was able to show successfully that hematoporphyrin could be used as a photosensitizer when exposed to light and oxygen in both guinea pigs and in mice. Meyer-Betz [5], in 1913, decided that it was necessary to study the hematoporphyrin in humans and since this had not been done before, he self-injected the photosensitizer into his own skin. What he noted was that when the injected areas were exposed to a light source, the areas injected became swollen and painful. And he observed that the phototoxic reaction that he was experiencing was not a self-limited one, in that the phototoxic reaction that he had been experiencing continued for 2 full months. Although hematoporphyrin is successful as a photosensitizer, the fact that it was not self-limiting made it difficult for clinicians of the day to use it on actual patients, and interest waned on how best to use PDT in everyday medicine and dermatology.

It was not until 1942 that interest once again with hematoporphyrin resurfaced in dermatology. Auler and Banzer [6] reported that hematoporphyrin was concentrating in certain dermatologic skin tumors and not in the surrounding structures around the tumors. They also noted that when the tumors were fluoresced with light, the tumors became necrotic over time, leaving the remaining skin normal. This again explained the uniqueness of PDT for use in medicine and for selective destruction of a target tissue in dermatology. Several years later, Figge et al. [7] reported their findings with the use of hematoporphyrin as a photosensitizer. They noted that hematoporphyrin could be selectively absorbed into other cells within the body, specifically embryonic cells, traumatized skin cells, and in certain neoplastic cells.

Table 1. Common uses of PDT in dermatology

Actinic keratoses
Photodamage with associated actinic keratoses
Actinic cheilitis
Bowen's disease
Superficial basal cell carcinoma
Superficial squamous cell carcinoma
Acne vulgaris
Sebaceous gland hyperplasia
Hidradenitis suppurativa
Human papillomavirus infection
Molluscum contagiosum
Psoriasis vulgaris
Alopecia areata
Hirsutism
Cutaneous T-cell lymphoma
Kaposi's sarcoma
Malignant melanoma
Keratoacanthoma

Common uses in the United States are italicized.

From these humble beginnings, the groundwork for the use of PDT in medicine, and specifically in dermatology, had been laid out for us to continue to study, evaluate, and work with photosensitizers that were easily available, easily applied to the skin, and would carry out the photodynamic reaction with minimal adverse events. That became the next challenge for the PDT researchers of the day. The principle of PDT, i.e. the use of a photosensitizer, which now became hematoporphyrin for dermatologic research, which was selectively absorbed into cancerous skin cells, could be activated by an appropriate light source, and, in the presence of oxygen, cause selective destruction of the cancerous cell.

The next major breakthrough in dermatologic research on PDT came in 1978, when Dougherty et al. [8] described a new photosensitizer, which became known as hematoporphyrin purified derivative (HPD). HPD was a complex of porphyrin subunits and porphyrin by-products. The group successfully demonstrated that HPD could be successfully used to treat cutaneous malignancies with an appropriate light source, which in this case was a red light source. This was an extremely important contribution to the PDT literature, and systemic HPD became the standard for PDT for the next 10 years of PDT. A variety of medical uses emerged for PDT during this period of time, both oncologic and nononcologic, and some of the more common indications for PDT use in dermatology are shown in table 1.

The skin is a great resource for medical research, especially PDT research, since exposure to both natural and artificial light sources can be done with relative ease. Interest in PDT as a potential therapy for many skin concerns continued to grow with the use of HPD. However, because HPD remained phototoxic on the skin for several

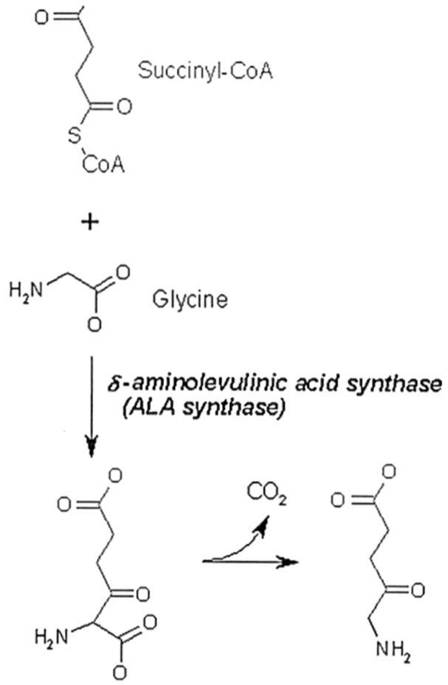

Fig. 1. The heme biosynthetic pathway. PpIX absorption in vivo (mouse skin). ALA is the natural precursor of PpIX in the heme pathway.

months as its precursor did, many did not favor its practical use. Then, in 1990, Kennedy et al. [9] introduced the first topical porphyrin derivative and the face of PDT changed forever. This topical porphyrin derivative was 5-aminolevulinic acid (ALA), and this would be the photosensitizer that would become the standard for PDT to this day.

ALA is known in medicine as a prodrug, which, when incorporated into a cell, is converted into its active drug form. Kennedy et al. [9] found that topical ALA could penetrate through the skin's main barrier, the stratum corneum, and once past the barrier, be absorbed selectively by actinically damaged skin cells, which opened the door for dermatologists to potentially treat actinic keratoses, becoming more and more prevalent in our society. They also noted that the topically applied ALA was selectively absorbed into nonmelanoma skin cells and also into the pilosebaceous units of the skin. They first described the PDT reaction with ALA. Once incorporated into the skin, ALA, which is a prodrug, is absorbed through the stratum corneum, enters the specific cells that are in the area, whether actinically damaged skin cells or nonmelanoma skin cells, or the pilosebaceous units, and is converted into its active form, which is known as protoporphyrin IX (PpIX).

In order to understand ALA and PpIX, one must look at the heme pathway, as shown in figure 1. ALA is the prodrug photosensitizing agent and PpIX is the actual photosensitizer. In order for the PDT reaction to be successful, the photosensitizer must be exposed to a light source with an appropriate wavelength that will interact with the photosensitizer. PpIX has been studied extensively with a variety of lasers and

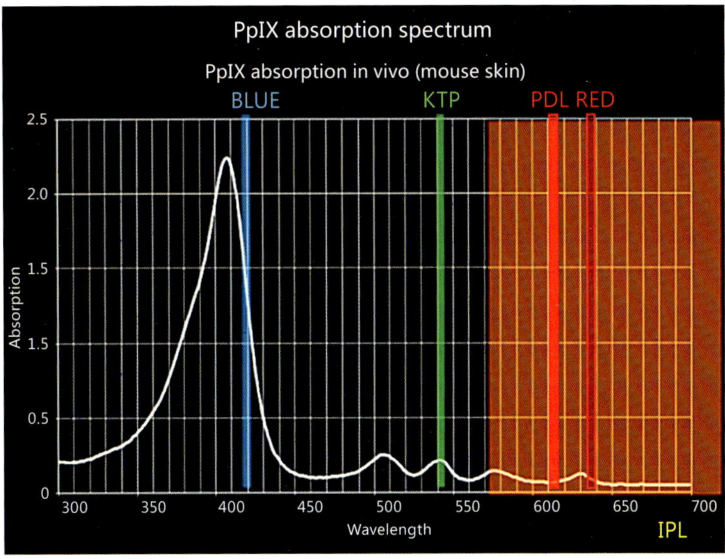

Fig. 2. The absorption spectrum of PpIX, and the lasers and light sources which have been shown to be useful in the activation of PpIX.

light sources over the past 35 years, and many of those devices will be described more in later chapters in this book. What should be noted here is that blue light has been the most studied light source in the United States, although many use blue light and other light sources routinely in their clinical practices.

The absorption spectrum of PpIX has been elucidated and is shown in figure 2 with the various lasers and light sources that can successfully activate PpIX. The peak absorption bands noted are in the blue light range, and these peaks are known as the Soret bands. Smaller peaks are also noted in the red light range, which is also very important for dermatologic applications of PDT. In Europe, the methyl ester of ALA, commonly referred to as methyl aminolevulinate (MAL), is the most common photosensitizer that is currently used, and a great deal of research with MAL and red light has been performed and will be reviewed later.

When one looks at the absorption spectrum of PpIX, one also notices several smaller peaks between blue and red light. These peaks have become important for many as certain lasers and light sources have been shown to work within these peaks to activate ALA or MAL, and have helped expand the use of PDT as we move further into the 21st century, a long road traveled since 1900 and our first foray into PDT.

One of the main advantages of using ALA or MAL for our current-day PDT use is that we have shortened tremendously the phototoxic reaction times of the drug on the skin. This has to do with the heme pathway, once again shown in figure 1. The heme biosynthetic pathway is maintained under a very close feedback loop system, which does not allow for the buildup of heme or any of its precursors, including PpIX in tissues. Exogenous ALA forming PpIX is cleared from the body much more rapidly than its predecessor HPD. Therefore, the potential for ALA to form a phototoxic skin reaction is considerably reduced as compared to HPD. We now note that this potential is only several days in most accounts as compared to the several months that were seen with HPD. And with the specificity that exists with ALA, this has become an ideal photosensitizer for dermatology.

PDT has taken two separate pathways into our dermatologic clinics, and this is a result of the manufacturing and production process that has emerged in the PDT world. In the United States, we have focused our attention on topical ALA, which commercially is a 20% ALA solution known as Levulan® Kerastick™, manufactured by DUSA Pharmaceuticals (Wilmington, Mass., USA). The only FDA indication, which will be explained later, is for the treatment of nonhyperkeratotic actinic keratoses of the face and scalp using a blue light source. Many clinicians utilize Levulan® off-label for a variety of indications, including moderate-to-severe acne vulgaris, sebaceous gland hyperplasia, hidradenitis suppurativa, and for nonmelanoma superficial skin cancers.

In Europe, research has centered primarily on MAL. It is commercially available as a 16.8% cream, known as Metvix®, from Galderma Laboratories (Fort Worth, Tex., USA). Its primary use in Europe has been in the treatment of nonmelanoma skin cancers with the use of red light as the main light source. Off-label, Metvix® has been used for the same indications as ALA in the United States [10]. MAL did have FDA approval for the use in the treatment of actinic keratoses with red light in the United States, but was never widely used and is no longer available at the time of this writing on the US market.

This textbook will explore PDT and its uses in dermatology today from a group of highly respected clinicians that have helped make PDT a common and an accepted form of therapy for our patients who benefit from our work. PDT is used and should be used daily in our dermatology practices, and we have gained much understanding of and insight into the past on how to best accomplish this. Looking ahead, we will continue to look at our photosensitizers and see if we can improve on them. We will continue to look at the light sources we use, and how we can maximize them, how we can combine them, and what the best approaches are when it comes to temperature and sunlight – whether daylight PDT has a significant role for us to consider moving forward. And as well, the concept of drug delivery is very important today, and how we can use lasers and light sources to help make the delivery of our photosensitizers better, all are under study, and will help shape the future of PDT for all of us.

PDT has become a truly global therapeutic modality that affects lives. The hope of this textbook is to bring all of you together – some of the brightest minds in PDT from all over the world – to share the science that exists and learn from the experiences made, to make this the most up-to-date review on PDT yet, and my sincere thanks to all of them.

References

1 Raab O: Über die Wirkung fluoreszierender Stoffe auf Infusorien. Z Biol 1900;39:524–526.

2 von Tappeiner H, Jodblauer A: Über die Wirkung der photodynamischen (fluoreszierenden) Stoffe auf Protozoen und Enzyme. Dtsch Arch Klin Med 1904; 80:427–487.

3 Jesionek A, von Tappeiner H: Zur Behandlung der Hautcarcinome mit fluoreszierenden Stoffen. Dtsch Arch Klin Med 1905;85:223–227.

4 Hausman W: Die sensibilisierende Wirkung des Hämatoporphyrins. Biochem Z 1911;30:276–316.

5 Meyer-Betz D: Untersuchungen über die biologische (photodynamische) Wirkung des Hämatoporphyrins und anderer Derivative des Blut- und Gallenfarbstoffs. Dtsch Arch Klin Med 1913;112:476–503.

6 Auler H, Banzer G: Untersuchungen über die Rolle der Porphyrine bei geschwulstkranken Menschen und Tieren. Z Krebsforsch 1942;53:65–68.

7 Figge FHJ, Weiland GS, Manganiello LDJ: Cancer detection and therapy. Affinity of neoplastic embryonic and traumatized tissue for porphyrins and metalloporphyrins. Proc Soc Exp Biol Med 1948;68:640.

8 Dougherty TJ, Kaufman JE, Goldfarb A, Weishaupt KR, Boyle D, Middleman A: Photoradiation therapy for the treatment of malignant tumors. Cancer Res 1978;38:2628–2635.

9 Kennedy JC, Pottier RH, Pross DC: Photodynamic therapy with endogenous protoporphyrin IX: basic principles and present clinical experiences. J Photochem Photobiol B 1990;6:143–148.

10 Gold MH, Goldman MP: 5-Aminolevulinic acid photodynamic therapy: where we have been and where we are going. Dermatol Surg 2004;30:1077–1084.

Michael H. Gold, MD
Gold Skin Care Center
Tennessee Clinical Research Center
2000 Richard Jones Road, Suite 220, Nashville, TN 37215 (USA)
E-Mail drgold@goldskincare.com

Gold MH (ed): Cosmetic Photodynamic Therapy. Aesthet Dermatol. Basel, Karger, 2016, vol 3, pp 8–35
DOI: 10.1159/000439328

Photodynamic Therapy in Treating Actinic Keratosis and Photorejuvenation

Jennifer D. Peterson[a] · Mitchel P. Goldman[b]

[a]Suzanne Bruce and Associates, Katy, Tex., and [b]Goldman, Butterwick, Fitzpatrick, Groff, and Fabi, San Diego, Calif., USA

Abstract

The first photosensitizer prodrug to be FDA approved for use in topical photodynamic therapy (PDT) was aminolevulinic acid (ALA). Studies investigating the treatment of nonhyperkeratotic actinic keratoses (AKs) with ALA-PDT have led to multiple advances and refinements in treatment over the last decade. Incubation times of ALA have decreased, multiple light sources have been used to elicit the reaction, and cosmetic benefits of treatment have been discovered. In the following chapter, the background of ALA-PDT will be reviewed and clinical studies regarding the treatment of AKs and photorejuvenation are summarized. Finally, a practical guide for ALA-PDT treatment is provided in order to optimize treatment while avoiding common pitfalls of treatment.

Introduction

The first photosensitizer prodrug to be FDA approved for use in topical photodynamic therapy (PDT) was 5-δ-aminolevulinic acid (ALA). Studies investigating the treatment of nonhyperkeratotic actinic keratoses (AKs) with ALA-PDT have led to multiple advances and refinements in treatment over the last decade. Incubation times of ALA have decreased, multiple light sources have been used to elicit the reaction, and cosmetic benefits of treatment have been discovered. In the following chapter, the background of ALA-PDT will be reviewed and clinical studies regarding the treatment of AKs and photorejuvenation are summarized. Finally, a practical guide for ALA-PDT is provided in order to optimize treatment while avoiding common pitfalls of treatment.

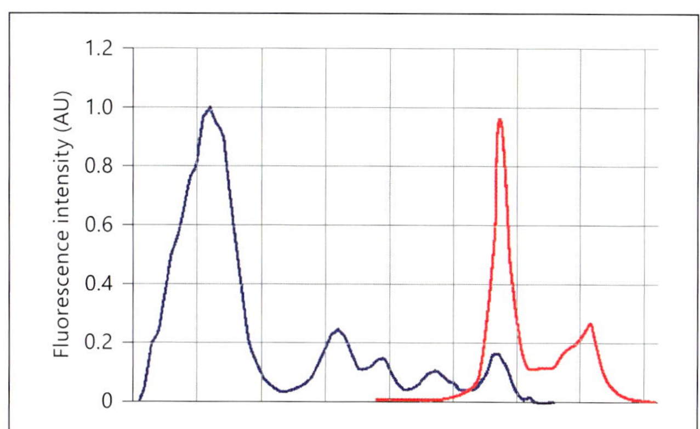

Fig. 1. Porphyrin absorption curve displays maximum absorption in the Soret band (360–400 nm) followed by 4 smaller peaks between 500 and 635 nm (Q bands). AU = Arbitrary units.

Background

The first topical porphyrin derivative, ALA, a natural precursor of protoporphyrin IX (PpIX) in the heme pathway, was introduced in 1999 by Kennedy et al. [1]. ALA acts as a prodrug-photosensitizing agent with the ability to penetrate the stratum corneum of the skin and be absorbed by actinically damaged skin cells and pilosebaceous units, whereas PpIX is the actual photosensitizer. Years later, a lipophilic ALA ester derivative, methyl aminolevulinate (MAL), was developed, showing stronger porphyrin fluorescence and better tumor selectivity, most likely because of enhanced penetration through cellular membranes compared with the hydrophilic ALA [2]. Recently, Ko et al. [3] showed no significant differences in complete response rates, recurrence rates, or cosmetic outcomes 12 months after PDT treatment of AKs with ALA or MAL; however, subjects reported ALA-PDT was more painful than MAL-PDT.

Mechanism of Action

Porphyrins exhibit a maximum absorption in the Soret band (360–400 nm) followed by 4 smaller peaks between 500 and 635 nm (Q bands; fig. 1) [4]. PDT involves the activation of a photosensitizer by light in the presence of an oxygen-rich environment. Topical PDT involves the application of ALA or MAL to the skin for some time, known as incubation time. This leads to the conversion of ALA to PpIX. PpIX accumulates in rapidly proliferating cells of premalignant and malignant lesions [5], as well as in blood vessels, melanin, and sebaceous glands [6]. Upon activation by a light source and in the presence of oxygen, the sensitizer (PpIX) is oxidized, a process called 'photobleaching' [7]. During this process, free radical oxygen singlets are generated, leading to selective destruction of tumor cells by apoptosis without collateral damage to surrounding tissues [8, 9].

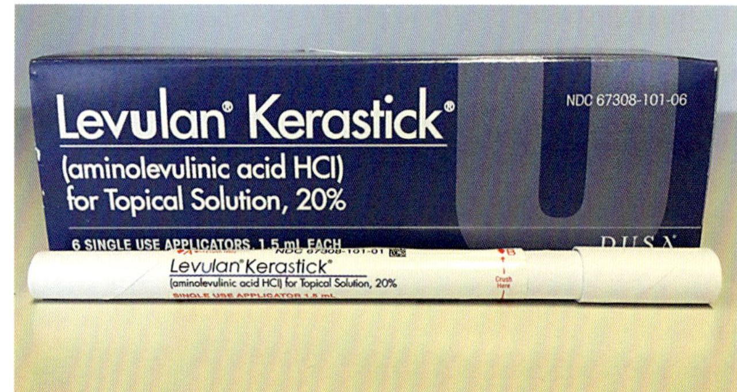

Fig. 2. In the US, ALA is available as a 20% topical solution manufactured under the name Levulan® Kerastick® (DUSA Pharmaceuticals).

Pharmacology

ALA is a hydrophilic, low-molecular-weight molecule within the heme biosynthesis pathway [5, 10]. In the US, ALA is available as a 20% topical solution manufactured under the name Levulan® Kerastick® (DUSA, Wilmington, Mass., USA; fig. 2). Since 1999, Levulan is FDA approved for the treatment of nonhyperkeratotic AKs on the face and scalp in conjunction with a blue light source, such as BluU (DUSA) [11]. It is supplied as a cardboard tube housing two sealed glass ampules, one containing 354 mg of ALA hydrochloride powder and the other 1.5 ml of solvent [12]. These separate components are mixed within the cardboard sleeve just prior to use.

Choice of Light Devices and Lasers

No standardized guidelines for the 'optimal irradiance, wavelength and total dose characteristics for PDT' exist according to the British Dermatology group and the American Society of Photodynamic Therapy Board [13–15]. However, certain laser and light sources are predictably chosen for PDT activation as their wavelengths correspond closely with the four absorption peaks along the porphyrin curve. The Soret band (400–410 nm), with a maximal absorption at 405–409 nm, is the highest peak along this curve for photoactivating PpIX. Smaller peaks designated as the 'Q bands' exist at approximately 505–510, 540–545, 580–584, and 630–635 nm [5, 6, 10]. There are advantages and disadvantages to exploiting the wavebands in either the Soret or Q bands for PDT. The Soret band peak is 10- to 20-fold larger than the Q bands, and blue light sources are often used to activate PpIX within this portion of the porphyrin curve, targeting lesions up to 2 mm in depth [16]. Longer wavelengths found within the Q bands produce a red light that penetrates more deeply (5 mm into the skin), but necessitate higher energy requirements [5, 10].

PDT light sources can be categorized in a variety of ways, including incoherent versus coherent sources, or by color (and wavelengths) emitted. Incoherent light is emitted as noncollimated light and is provided through broadband lamps, light-emitting diodes (LEDs), and intense pulsed light (IPL) systems. Incoherent light sources are easy to use, affordable, easily obtained, and portable due to their compact size [17]. Lasers provide precise doses of light radiation. As a collimated light source, lasers deliver energy to target tissues at specific wavelengths chosen to mimic absorption peaks along the porphyrin curve. Lasers used in PDT include the tunable argon dye laser (blue-green light, 450–530 nm) [18], the copper vapor laser-pumped dye laser (510–578 nm), long-pulsed dye lasers (PDLs; 585–595 nm), the Nd:YAG KTP dye laser (532 nm), the gold vapor laser (628 nm), and solid-state diode lasers (630 nm) [19].

Actinic Keratoses

Therapeutic Strategies

Given the premalignant potential of AKs, early treatment is paramount to preventing disease progression. Treatment options for AKs depend on a variety of factors including severity of involvement, duration or persistence of lesions, patient tolerability or desire for cosmesis, affordability/insurance coverage, and physician comfort with available treatment modalities [20, 21]. While solitary or few lesions may be approached with localized treatments such as cryotherapy, curettage, excision, or dermabrasion, field treatment may be more appropriate when numerous lesions are identified. Field therapy has the advantage of simultaneously treating subclinical AKs. Chemical peels, laser resurfacing, 5-fluorouracil (5-FU), topical diclofenac, topical retinoids, and topical immunomodulators (imiquimod) are all reasonable field treatment options in addition to PDT.

A comparison of PDT to other field treatment options for AKs yields comparable clearance rates [22, 23]. In fact, a comparison of 100% clearance rates from phase III clinical trials reported complete AK clearance with ALA-PDT in 72%, comparable to 5-FU (72%), and superior to imiquimod (49%) and diclofenac (48%) [24]. A direct comparison study by Kurwa et al. [25] found comparable lesion area reduction rates between ALA-PDT (73%) and 5-FU (70%). A recent meta-analysis evaluating AK clearance found 5-FU to be superior to PDT though PDT was felt to have similar results to imiquimod and ingenol mebutate. Finally, PDT was found to be more effective than cryotherapy or diclofenac [26].

Therapy Advantages/Disadvantages

Clearance rates of AKs following PDT have ranged from 68 to 98% [27, 28]. Assuming near equivalent or even superior clearance rates of PDT compared to other field treatment options, PDT has several advantages in the treatment of AKs. Improvement of photodamage, superior cosmesis, and better patient satisfaction were documented in multiple studies [23, 28]. Other procedures used for the clearance of AKs such as cryotherapy or chemical peels can result in hypopigmentation or even scarring [23, 29]. PDT, perhaps surprisingly to some, is a cost-effective means of treating AKs. Gold [24] found ALA-PDT with a blue light source to be the least expensive treatment option for AKs compared to 5-FU, imiquimod, and diclofenac. In fact, ALA-PDT was approximately one half the costs of a similar course of imiquimod for field AK treatment.

Disadvantages of PDT are largely related to minor and expected adverse events following the procedure. Minor pain and erythema may occur during or following the procedure. Mild crusting and edema may occur, lasting up to 1 week. However, other treatment modalities for AKs have similar if not longer recovery periods. There are financial costs associated with the procedure. If PDT is performed for AK treatment and photorejuvenation, there is an associated out-of-pocket cost to the patient. The physician must also make an initial investment in the laser and light devices, although many of the light sources have multiple applications beyond PDT.

Treatment Results Organized by Light Source

A variety of light sources have been investigated for use in PDT for the treatment of AKs; therefore, we have organized clinical studies according to the most common light sources available. Table 1 provides a summary of peer-reviewed articles on the use of ALA-PDT in AK treatment.

Blue Light

Perhaps the most popular emission spectrum utilized in the US, blue light, was the first FDA-approved form of light for activating ALA (fig. 3). As the relatively shorter wavelength of blue light only penetrates 1–2 mm, but is potent in its photochemical effect, blue light is often selected for the treatment of superficial lesions such as non-hyperkeratotic AK lesions [30]. In 2001, Jeffes et al. [22] reported the usage of ALA-PDT with a 14- to 18-hour incubation using blue light (417 nm) to AKs of the face and scalp in 36 patients. Light exposure duration was 16 min and 40 s, now considered standard treatment. Eight weeks following a single treatment, 88% of lesions cleared. A similarly designed study of 64 patients [31] displayed 75% or more clearance of AK lesions following one treatment. However, 14% of patients required reduced power density during blue light irradiation due to intolerable side effects including stinging and burning.

In a large study of 243 subjects, Piacquadio et al. [32] found a 70% complete clearance 12 weeks following one PDT session. A second treatment resulted in a complete clearance rate of 88%. Facial lesions responded more favorably than scalp lesions, with complete response rates of 78 and 50%, respectively, 12 weeks following treatment; 94% of subjects evaluated their cosmetic outcome following PDT as good or excellent. Recurrence for this treatment cohort 8–12 weeks after treatment was 5% [31].

Table 1. Published clinical studies on ALA-PDT for AKs

First author, year	ALA preparation	Location of AKs	Incubation period, h	Lesions treated (patients), n	Light source (wavelength, nm)	Response rate	Follow-up, months
Kennedy [1], 1990	20% emulsion	Not specified	3–6		Tungsten (>600)	90% CR	18
Wolf [9], 1993	20% emulsion	Face, scalp	4–8	9	Tungsten, unfiltered	100% CR	3–12
Morton [81], 1995	20% emulsion	Face, scalp	4	4	Xenon (630)	100% CR	12
Fijan [82], 1995	20% emulsion	Not specified	20, occluded	43 (9)	Halogen (570–690)	81% CR	3–20
Szeimies [83], 1996	10% emulsion	Head, hands, arms	6, occluded	36 (10)	Waldmann red lamp (580–740)	71% CR head	1
Fink-Puches [84], 1997	20% emulsion	Head, neck, forearms, dorsal hands	4, occluded	251 (28)	Halogen slide projector (300–800) with cutoff filters at 515, 530, 570, 610	71% CR	36
Fritsch [85], 1997	10% ointment	Face, scalp	6, occluded	(6)	Green lamp (543–548) vs. red Waldmann lamp (570–750)	100% CR for both green and red light	15
Jeffes et al. [71], 1997	0–30% emulsion	Face, scalp, trunk, extremities	3, occluded	240 (40)	Argon dye laser (630)	91% CR face/scalp; 45% CR trunk/extremities	2
Karrer et al. [86], 1999	20% emulsion	Scalp, face	6, occluded	200 (24)	Red light lamp (580–740) or PDL (585)	84% CR (red light) 79% CR (PDL)	1
Kurwa et al. [25], 1999	20% emulsion	Hands	4, occluded	(14)	Metal halide lamp (580–740)	73% lesion area reduction; comparable to 5-FU	6
Itoh [36], 2000	20% emulsion, 2 or more sessions	Face, neck, extremities	4, occluded	53 (10)	Red lamp (peak 630, range 600–700), excimer dye laser (630)	82% CR face/neck; 56% CR extremities	12
Dijkstra [87], 2001	20% gel, 2 sessions	Unspecified	8, occluded	4	Violet lamp (400–450)	50% CR	3–12
Jeffes [22], 2001	20% solution	Face, scalp	14–18	70 (36)	Blue light (417)	85% CR	4
Markam [46], 2001	Concentration unspecified, cream	Scalp	4, occluded	(4)	Red light (580–740)	75% CR	6

Table 1. Continued

First author, year	ALA preparation	Location of AKs	Incubation period, h	Lesions treated (patients), n	Light source (wavelength, nm)	Response rate	Follow-up, months
Varma [37], 2001	20% ointment	Not specified	4, occluded	127 (88 patients with mixed diagnoses)	Waldmann red lamp (580–740)	77% CR after 1st, 99% after 2nd, RR of 28%	6
Ruiz–Rodriguez [56], 2002	20% emulsion	Face, scalp	4, occluded	38	IPL (590–1,200)	76% CR 1 session; 91% CR 2 sessions	3
Alexiades–Armenakas [29], 2003	20% solution	Head, trunk extremities	3 with occlusion; 14–18 without occlusion	3,622 (36)	Long-PDL (595)	90–100% CR	8
Clark [19], 2003	20% ointment	Not specified	4	23	Metal halide (590–730); halogen lamp (570–680); diode laser (630)	91% CR	11
Goldman [28], 2003	20% solution	Face; long-incubation PDT	15–20	(32)	Blue light (417)	94% CR of AKs; improved skin texture, pigmentation	3–6
Smith [35], (2003)	20% solution, 2 sessions	Face, scalp	1	(35)	Blue light (417) or PDL (595)	80% CR for blue light; 60% CR for PDL	1
Dragieva [54], 2004	20% emulsion; transplant patients	Face, scalp	5, occluded	32 (20)	Red light (580–740)	94% CR at 4 weeks; 72% at 48 weeks	12
Piacquadio [32], 2004	20% solution, 1–2 sessions	Face, scalp	14–18	1,402 (243)	Blue (417)	91% CR 1 session; 83% CR 2 sessions	3
Touma [12], 2004	20% solution	Face	1–3	(17)	Blue lamp (417)	87–94% CR	5
Gilbert [41], 2005	20% solution, 5-FU daily × 5 days pre-PDT	Face	0.5–0.75	(15)	IPL (560–1,200)	90% CR with combination therapy	12
Kim [40], 2005	20% emulsion	Face	4, occluded	12 (7)	IPL (555–950)	50%	3
Tschen [73], 2006	20% solution, 1–2 treatment sessions	Face, scalp	14–18	968 (110)	Blue (417)	72–76% CR 1 session; 86% 2 sessions	12

Table 1. Continued

First author, year	ALA preparation	Location of AKs	Incubation period, h	Lesions treated (patients), n	Light source (wavelength, nm)	Response rate	Follow-up, months
Calzavara-Pinton [5], 2007	20% cream	Face	6–8	50 (from a pool of 85 patients with AKs, BCCs, SCCs, Bowen's disease)	Argon dye laser (630)	100% CR	24–36
Nakano [15], 2009	20% cream (3 treatment sessions)	Face	4, occluded	(30)	Excimer dye laser (630 nm)	100% CR in lesions <10 mm; 70% CR in lesions >10 mm in diameter	12
Taub [33], 2011	20% solution	Hands, forearms	2, occluded	Not listed (15)	Blue (417 nm)	58.4% reduction in lesion count	1
Schmieder [34], 2012	20% solution	Dorsal hands, forearms	3, occluded vs. unoccluded	182 (70)	Blue (417 nm)	88.7% reduction in lesion count if occluded; 70% unoccluded	3
Jang [45], 2013	20% solution	Face	70–90 min	34 (29)	Fractionated CO_2 (10,600 nm) followed by red (600–720 nm)	70.6%	6
Tanaka [44], 2013	20% solution	Face	Not reported	40 (18)	Excimer dye (630 nm)	100% CR with ALA + imiquimod; 41.7% ALA; 66.7% imiquimod	1
Cai [88], 2013	20% solution	Face	5, occluded	56 (42)	Red (630 nm)	85.71% CR	1
Willey [52], 2014	20% solution	Upper or lower extremities	1, occluded and one side heated with heating pad on medium	275 (20)	Blue (417 nm)	Without heat: 67.5% CR; With heat: 88% CR	6
Ko [3], 2014	20% solution ALA or 16% MAL cream	Face	ALA: 6, MAL: 3; both occluded	222 (58)	ALA: halogen (nm); MAL: red (630 nm)	56.9% CR for ALA; 50.7% for MAL	12

BCCs = Basal cell carcinomas; CR = complete response; RR = recurrence rate at 12 months; SCCs = squamous cell carcinomas.

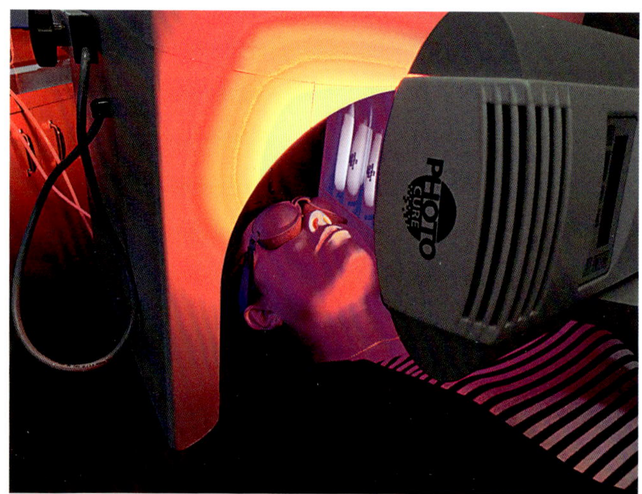

Fig. 3. Noncoherent blue lamp is a common choice for photoactivating ALA in the US. The BluU (DUSA Pharmaceuticals) emits light at a bandwidth of approximately 417 ± 5 nm. Red light (Aktilite; Galderma, Fort Worth, Tex., USA) emits light at a bandwidth of approximately 630 ± 40 nm and is FDA approved for activation of Medvixia. During our illumination, we simultaneously deliver blue and red light. The patient is placed directly under the blue light with the red light placed at the outlet of the blue light.

The efficacy of PDT is reduced when treating AKs on the extremities. Taub and Garretson [33] found two ALA-PDT treatments using a 2-hour occluded incubation followed by blue light activation resulted in a 58.4% reduction in lesion counts at 1 month. Schmieder et al. [34] performed a larger study on the dorsal hands and forearms of 70 subjects, and compared the efficacy and side effects of occlusion versus nonocclusion of ALA during a 3-hour incubation. The majority (83%) of subjects received two treatments, while the remainder received a single treatment. Lesion counts at 6 months were reduced by 88.7% when ALA was occluded and 70% if not occluded. Postprocedural erythema and edema were more prominent and common following ALA-PDT occlusion.

Multiple studies have demonstrated a reduction in AKs in addition to photorejuvenative effects on the treated areas of the skin [28, 31]. In 2004, Touma et al. [12] reported on the efficacy of short-contact ALA-PDT. Not only did this allow for PDT to be conducted in a single clinic visit rather than over 2 days, side effects were also reduced. Clearance rates of 93, 84, and 90% were achieved in the 1-, 2-, and 3-hour incubation groups, respectively, and were maintained through the 5-month follow-up. In addition, the subjects in this study also showed a modest, but significant improvement in photoaging.

Yellow-Orange Light – Pulsed Dye Laser

Long-PDLs (585–595 nm) target the chromophore oxyhemoglobin, allowing selective destruction of blood vessels. As AKs often appear as erythematous scaly plaques, the inflammatory nature of these lesions can be targeted with this vascular laser. Alexiades-Armenakas and Geronemus [29] were the first to report on its use in ALA-PDT. Thirty-six patients and a total of 3,622 lesions (face and scalp – 2,620, extremities –

949, and trunk – 53) were treated. ALA was applied with either a 3-hour, unoccluded incubation versus a 14- to 18-hour incubation. No difference in clearance was observed between the two incubation time groups. Clearance rates were highest for head lesions at 100%. According to this large cohort study, it appeared that PDL at subpurpuric doses allows an efficient and less painful means of accomplishing PDT. Smith et al. [35] found AK clearance rates were similar to those of topical 5-FU or ALA-PDL (79 vs. 80%), but clearance rate of PDT using a blue light source was lower (60%). Additionally, improvements in global photodamage, hyperpigmentation, and tactile roughness were also observed.

Red Light

The longer wavelength of red light allows deeper tissue penetration, up to 5 mm. Red light is used frequently during PDT with MAL; however, it may also be used for photoactivation of PpIX during ALA-PDT. Wavelengths in the red light spectrum, usually targeted around 630 nm, can be emitted by an argon pumped dye laser, excimer laser, metal halide lamps, and red LED lamps.

Several studies have reported clearance rates of facial AKs between 71 and 99%. Kurwa et al. [25] used a metal halide lamp for ALA-PDT to treat the dorsal hands, resulting in a 79.5% decrease in AKs lesions. Itoh et al. [36] treated Japanese patients with AKs on the face, neck, and extremities. With two or more treatments, clearance rates at 12 months were higher for lesions on the head and neck (81.8%) compared to the extremities (55.6%). One possible explanation for an increased resistance of AKs of the extremities would be the lack of pilosebaceous units in these areas, which are important for a better absorption of prodrug and so to a better response. No serious adverse effects were reported in these patients with darker skin types. Research by Varma et al. [37] found complete clearance rates for AKs after one and two treatments were 77 and 99%, respectively. However, the recurrence rate at 12 months was 28%. Moseley et al. [38] demonstrated a 92% AK clearance rate after 2 treatments, with 100% clearance after three ALA-PDT sessions.

Intense Pulsed Light

IPL devices emit noncollimated, noncoherent light with wavelengths in the range of 515–1,200 nm, which corresponds to the visible light and near-infrared spectrum [39]. Various filters can be used to block certain wavelengths below the cutoff point of the desired filter. The light source is particularly useful in photorejuvenation, targeting hyperpigmentation, blood vessels, and collagen. A small study by Kim et al. [40] documented the use of ALA-IPL for the treatment of AKs exclusively. Twelve facial AK lesions in 7 patients treated with a single session of ALA-PDT showed a 50% clearance rate at the 12-week follow-up. This clearance rate is markedly lower than reported averages, but it is difficult to formulate sound conclusions based on the small sample size. Further studies evaluating the simultaneous improvement in AKs and photorejuvenation are discussed below.

Several small case studies have demonstrated a possible synergistic effect of ALA-PDT with other treatment options for AKs. Gilbert [41] investigated 15 patients with multiple AKs treated with a 5-day course of nightly 5-FU cream to the face followed by short-contact PDT activated by an IPL source. A clearance rate of 90% was observed at the 1-year follow-up. Martin [42] performed a split-area study with 3 patients treated with ALA-PDT alone versus sequential therapy with 5-FU (7–10 days) and short-contact ALA-PDT (1-hour ALA incubation followed by blue light illumination at 417–432 nm). Six months after the initial visit, the combined regimen showed enhanced efficacy in treating AKs, suggesting synergistic effects of 5-FU and ALA-PDT.

Shaffelburg [43] conducted a split-face study of 24 patients with multiple AKs, in which ALA-PDT was performed on the entire face. One half of the face was also randomized to receive additional subsequent treatment with a 12-week regimen of imiquimod. Clearance rates at 12 months were superior on the combination treatment side, with 89.9% complete lesion clearance compared to 74.5% on the ALA-PDT side alone. In a three-arm study, Tanaka et al. [44] treated patients with either ALA alone, 5% imiquimod cream alone, or a combination of both. One month after treatment, 100% clearance was seen in the combination therapy. However, ALA-PDT alone achieved complete clearance rates in 41.7% and imiquimod cream in 66.7%. Finally, combination laser therapy utilizing ablative fractional laser therapy for drug delivery of ALA has been shown to decrease incubation time associated with ALA-PDT [45].

Clinical Technique and Treatment Protocol

Skin Preparation

Optimal results following ALA-PDT can be achieved with proper skin preparation prior to the procedure itself. The stratum corneum is a major barrier to the penetration of ALA [20, 31]. Hyperkeratotic lesions must be treated with light curettage prior to ALA application. Otherwise, ALA is preferentially absorbed by the hyperkeratotic scale rather than the lesion intended for treatment [46]. Some physicians use occlusion to improve delivery of ALA through thicker lesions and for lesions on the extremities. Schmieder et al. [34] found occlusion of ALA on the dorsal hands and forearms improved AK clearance rates to 88.7% with occlusion versus 70% without occlusion. Tegaderm™, opaque Mepore®, or Glad Press'n Seal® may be used for these purposes.

Methods of proper skin preparation to reduce stratum corneum thickness also include light chemical peels, tape stripping, microdermabrasion, oscillating sonic cleansing brushes (Clarisonic, Redmond, Wash., USA), and degreasing of the skin with acetone [14, 47–49]. All of the above measures can improve the absorption of ALA by the skin [50]. We routinely use a vibrating microdermabrasion system (Vibraderm, Great Plains, Tex., USA) with subsequent acetone degreasing to prepare the skin for ALA application.

Preoperative Considerations

Patients with a history of herpes simplex virus are prophylactically treated with oral antivirals. One week prior to PDT, patients are asked to discontinue the usage of topical retinoids, and α- and β-hydroxy acids, and to avoid chemical peels 1 month prior.

We do not routinely use topical or intralesional anesthesia prior to ALA-PDT. With a 1-hour incubation time, in our clinical experience, the procedure is well tolerated by the overwhelming majority of patients. We use forced air cooling and refrigerated conductive gel during the IPL portion of photoactivation, and a cooling fan with aerosolized water during blue light exposure. For longer incubation periods, the use of oral analgesics, topical lidocaine preparations, and ice packs in conjunction with PDT may increase patient comfort [28]. Borelli et al. [51] recently examined the effects of subcutaneous infiltration anesthesia (SIA) on pain in PDT. They compared the pain related to ALA-PDT in 16 patients who received oral analgesics (1 g paracetamol and 20 mg codeine) and SIA on one side of the face, containing a mixture of ropivacaine, prilocaine, and epinephrine. Significantly less pain was reported by 94% of the SIA patients. However, SIA should not contain vasoconstrictors, such as epinephrine, as their use could reduce the oxygen supply in the skin and thus compromise the effectiveness of PDT.

Incubation Time

ALA is FDA approved for use with a 14- to 18-hour incubation and subsequent photoactivation with blue light [11]. However, longer incubation times often result in an increased severity of adverse effects following ALA-PDT [22], and, furthermore, shorter incubation times (1–3 h) have demonstrated similar efficacy in AK clearance [12, 35]. We routinely use a 60-min incubation time in the treatment of AKs or for photorejuvenation. When treating thicker, larger, or more invasive lesions, we extend the incubation time to 3 h and occlude the treated area with Glad Press'n Seal®. Additionally, on the extremities, we incubate using occlusion [34] and simultaneous application of heating pads, set on low setting, to encourage the conversion of PpIX and improve efficacy [52].

Illumination

Blue, red, yellow-orange, and broadband light sources may be used to activate PpIX during ALA-PDT for AKs or photorejuvenation. It is our practice, both in the treatment of AKs and photorejuvenation, to use multiple light sources during ALA-PDT. With a typical treatment, we treat individual lesions first with subpurpuric doses of PDL, followed by full-face treatment by IPL, and, lastly, illumination with a blue and/or red light source. It should be noted that the IPL also results in hair reduction, so judicious use should be exercised in hair-bearing areas such as the scalp and beard area. In table 2, our treatment protocol for ALA-PDT is summarized [6]. This is supplied as an example, but is by no means the only way to successfully perform PDT. This may be used as a general guideline, and practitioners must

Table 2. Our clinical technique of ALA-PDT for facial AKs and photorejuvenation

ALA-PDT for facial AKs and photorejuvenation

1 Cleanse the patient's skin with mild soap and water

2 Perform microdermabrasion over the treated area
If a microdermabrasion system is unavailable, consider using an oscillating skin brush (Clarisonic Pro; Clarisonic, Redmond, Wash., USA) on high setting for 2 min while cleansing the skin

3 Scrub the skin vigorously using a 4 × 4 inch acetone-soaked gauze

4 Break the two glass ampules in the Levulan Kerastick as per the package insert [27]; shake the stick for about 2 min

5 Apply the ALA solution to the treatment area; this is best accomplished using a painting motion across the skin surface; at least two coats of the solution are recommended, and the entire contents of the Kerastick should be used; it is important to get close to the eyes, otherwise it will be apparent that the periorbital skin was not treated

6 Allow the Levulan to incubate for 60 min on the skin; the patient should remain indoors and away from sunlight during the incubation period

7 Remove the Levulan prior to any light treatment by requesting the patient to wash his/her face with a gentle soap and water

8 Activate the Levulan with the appropriate light source(s):

- A Illumination is begun with PDL to individual lesions (if PDL unavailable, proceed to IPL)
  - 1 595 nm, 7-mm spot size, 40-ms pulse width, and 10–12 J/cm^2 (Cynergy; Cynosure, Westford, Mass., USA) with forced cold air cooling
  - 2 595 nm, 7-mm spot size, 40-ms pulse width, dynamic cooling 30/30, and 10–12 J/cm^2 (Vbeam Perfecta; Candela, Irvine, Calif., USA)
- B Next, an IPL is utilized in non-hair-bearing areas
  - 1 For skin types I–III, we use the 560-nm cutoff filter and the 590-nm filter for skin types IV (Lumenis M22; Lumenis Ltd., Yokneam, Israel)
    - a If predominant hyperpigmentation: double pulse technique, 3.0-ms pulse duration for each pulse
    - b If combination of hyperpigmentation and erythema: double pulse technique, 3.5-ms pulse duration for each pulse
    - c Predominance of fine telangiectasias: double pulse technique, 4-ms pulse duration for each pulse
  - 2 10- to 30-ms delay is set between pulses in skin types I–III and 30–40 ms in skin type IV, increase delay for nonfacial locations
  - 3 Fluence range of 17–22 J/cm^2, with decreased fluences recommended for nonfacial locations
  - 4 Other IPL devices can also be used successfully, though treatment settings *must* be adjusted appropriately to each device
- C Finally, simultaneous illumination with blue and red light (fig. 3)
  - 1 Blue light source (BluU; DUSA Pharmaceuticals) positioned 25–50 mm from the skin, 16 min 40 s, light dose 10 J/cm^2
  - 2 Red light source (Aktilite CL 128; Galderma, Fort Worth, Tex., USA) positioned 50–80 mm from the skin, 8 min 49 s, 37 J/cm^2

9 Mineral-based sunscreen is applied and patient is discharged home

10 Instruct the patient on strict photoprotection for the following 36 h; the patient is to remain indoors, out of direct sunlight or bright indoor lights

11 Patients are provide a bland, ceramide-based cream to apply to their skin 4–6 times a day

12 Repeat the treatment in 4–8 weeks; if there was little reaction, increase the incubation time, reevaluate your skin preparation technique, or consider combination therapy

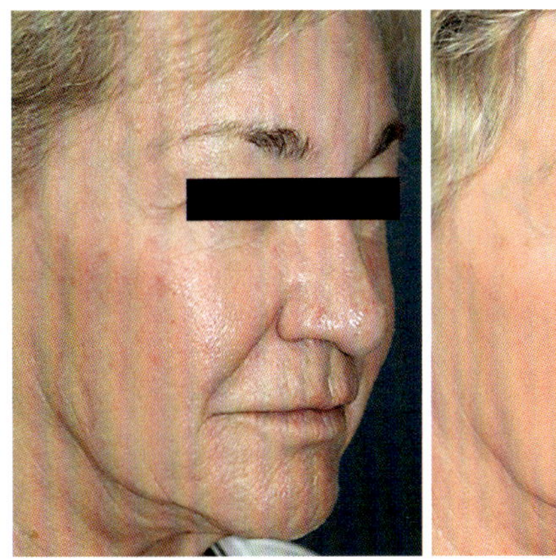
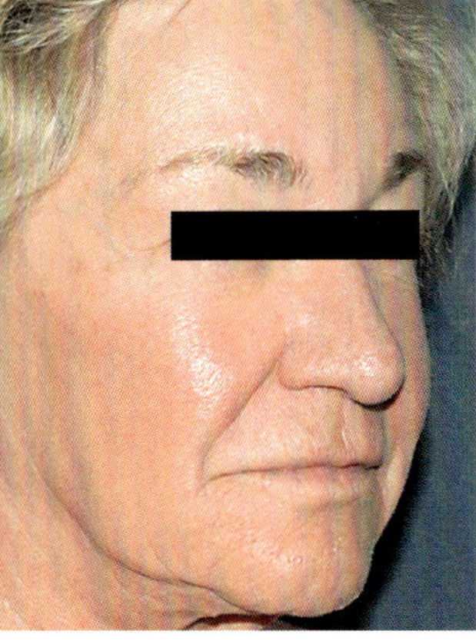

Fig. 4. Multiple AKs and extensive photodamage on the face of a female patient before and after one treatment of multilaser PDT utilizing PDL, IPL, and blue and red lights. Device settings are as follows: PDL (7-mm spot, 40-ms pulse duration, 11 J/cm^2), and IPL (560 nm crystal, double pulsed with a 4-ms pulse width and 20-ms pulse delay at 18 J/cm^2) and simultaneous illumination with blue light for 15 min and red light for 9 min. Note the improvement in the presence of AKs, solar lentigines, sallowness, and skin texture.

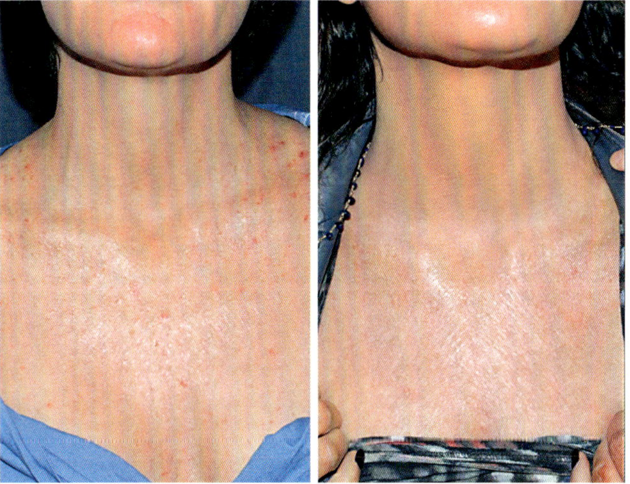

Fig. 5. Significant improvement in AKs on the chest of a middle-aged female following ALA-PDT to the chest.

decide for themselves the most effective and efficient use of ALA-PDT in their office. Clinical examples of AKs treated with a multilaser PDT approach are presented in figures 4–6.

Postoperative Considerations

Immediately following treatment, we apply a cooled, bland, gentle skin cream to the treated skin to calm erythema and irritation. A sunblock (physical blocker) containing zinc oxide and titanium dioxide is applied to the treated skin. To avoid

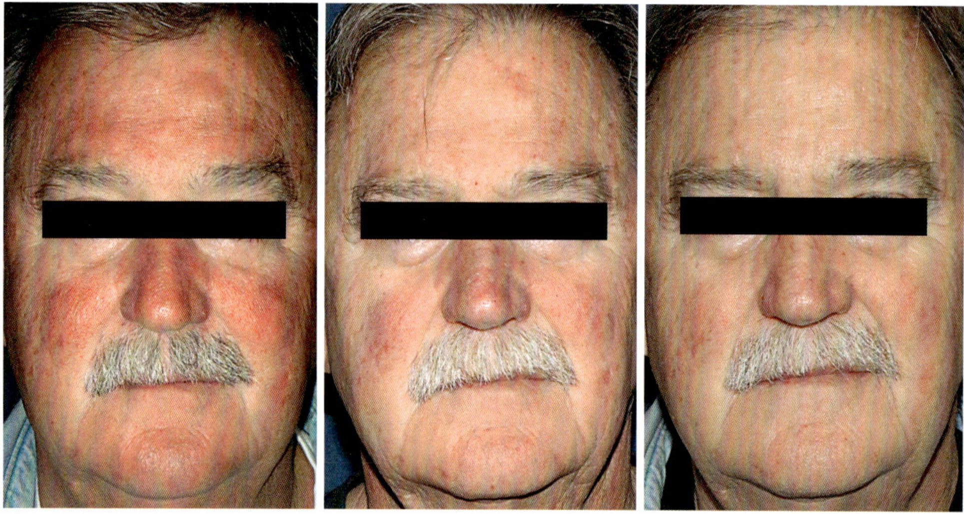

Fig. 6. Before and following a single treatment with multilaser PDT to the face of a male patient with reduction in AKs along with improvement in signs of photoaging and rosacea. Our multilaser PDT protocol involves sequential activation with PDL (7-mm spot, 40-ms pulse duration, 12 J/cm^2), intense PDL to non-hair-bearing areas (560 nm crystal; double pulsed with 4-ms pulse width and 20-ms pulse delay at 17 J/cm^2), and simultaneous illumination with blue (15 min) and red (9 min) lights.

phototoxicity during daylight hours, our patients are scheduled for treatment in the late afternoon, so they may depart the clinic during twilight hours. Patients are asked to wear sunglasses and protective clothing during their ride home.

We instruct patients to avoid sunlight and bright indoor light sources [18] for 36 h following treatment. We request our patients to return to the clinic 1 week and 2 months following PDT for routine follow-up. We perform subsequent rounds of ALA-PDT at 1- to 2-month intervals, and counsel patients to anticipate two to three ALA-PDT sessions for the treatment of AKs. These recommendations are consistent with consensus guidelines from the American Society of Photodynamic Therapy [13].

Special Considerations in Solid Organ Transplant Recipients

Solid organ transplant recipients (OTRs) suffer from a 10- to 250-fold increase in AKs due to their ongoing immunosuppressive therapy. In addition, the precancerous and cancerous lesions developing in the OTR population are often more aggressive [53], requiring frequent and ongoing cancer surveillance. Although initial response rates of AKs following PDT were comparable in the OTR patient population compared to normal controls [54], longer-term follow-up demonstrated statistically significant decreases in clearance rates in the OTR population. In addition, squamous cell carcinomas of the dorsal hands and forearms were not prevented in OTRs in a 2-year follow-up study, although there was a trend toward decreased keratotic regions in the areas treated [55]. PDT may still be a viable treatment option in this population, but it may

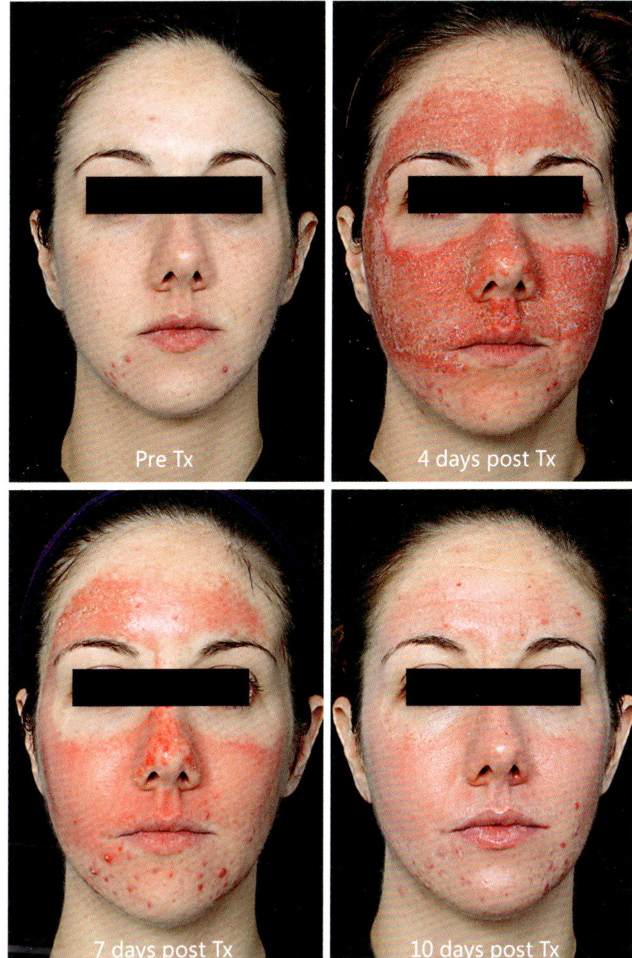

Fig. 7. Healing progression over 10 days in a young adult female following ALA-PDT. Erythema and edema predominate in the first 2–3 days, followed by crusting and peeling, which resolve in most instances within 1–2 weeks. Tx = Therapy.

require adjustments to typical treatment protocols including increased frequency of PDT sessions [54] and use of longer wavelengths (red light) for deeper skin penetration [55].

Photorejuvenation

Photoaging of the skin results from a combination of collective damage from ultraviolet exposure and the intrinsic aging process. Not only can the appearance be concerning to the patient, it can also lead to precancerous conditions with the development of AKs [56]. Photodamaged skin is characterized by skin laxity, lines/wrinkles, hyperpigmentation, sallowness, erythema, tactile roughness, atrophy, and telangiectasias [17].

Many of the same lasers and light sources effective in ALA-PDT for the treatment of AKs have the added benefit of inducing photorejuvenative effects on the skin. As mentioned previously, chromophores targeted during PDT may include vessels, melanin, and collagen [57]. Blue light only allows for a photochemical effect in PDT with less tissue penetration than other light sources such as IPL and PDL. The latter sources penetrate deeply enough to target vessels, pigment, and collagen [47]. The choice of which light source to use for ALA-PDT ultimately depends on such factors as the condition being treated, efficacy, cost of use, and availability of equipment.

Efficacy of Aminolevulinic Acid Combined with Photodynamic Therapy

Studies relating to the treatment of photodamage with ALA-PDT are organized in the following according to the light source employed. A summary of these studies is provided in table 3.

Blue Light

Despite the shallow penetration of blue light, it still appears to improve the signs of photoaging following ALA-PDT. The first indication that blue light had photorejuvenative effects in PDT was with the phase II/III clinical trials for FDA approval of Levulan for nonhyperkeratotic AKs where significant improvement in the signs of photoaging were noted after treatment [22, 32, 58]. Goldman and Atkin [28] utilized a single session of ALA-PDT (1-hour occlusion) with a blue light source in 32 patients. They found 72% improvement in skin texture and 59% improvement in skin pigmentation. Touma et al. [12] studied the effectiveness of ALA (short contact, 1–3 h) and blue light illumination in the treatment of AKs and diffuse photodamage. At 1- and 5-month follow-up intervals, there was not only a significant reduction in AKs, but also marked improvement in photodamage parameters such as skin quality, fine wrinkling, and sallowness. However, pigmentary changes and coarse wrinkling showed little to no improvement.

The study by Smith et al. [35], discussed earlier in this chapter, compared topical, low-concentration 5-FU to two forms of short-contact ALA-PDT: one arm with activation from a blue light source and the other with PDL. While 1 patient in the 5-FU group discontinued due to a confluent erythematous reaction, all patients in the ALA-PDT group completed the study. In both ALA-PDT groups, patients experienced improvement in global photodamage, hyperpigmentation, and tactile roughness. The ALA-PDL therapy was more successful in treating pigmentation and the ALA-blue light therapy had lower response rates to global photoaging.

Red Light

A histological and immunohistochemical analysis conducted by Park et al. [59] with ALA-PDT (twice at 1-month intervals, using red light at 580–740 nm, dose of 100 J/cm^2/100 mW/cm^2) showed significant increase in type I and III procollagen expression. Elastotic material with fibrilin-1 and tropoelastin expression in the dermis

Table 3. Published clinical studies on ALA-PDT for photorejuvenation

First author, year	ALA preparation	Location of photodamage/ study design	Incubation period, h	Patients, n	Light source (emission λ, nm)	Response	Follow-up, months
Ruiz-Rodriguez [56], 2002	20% emulsion	Face, scalp ≥1 AK and chronic photodamage; 2 PDT sessions	4, occluded	17 (38 AKs)	IPL (590–1,200)	87% CR of AKs; excellent cosmesis	3
Goldman [28], 2003	20% solution	Face, long-incubation PDT	15–20	32	Blue light (417)	94% CR of AKs; improved skin texture, pigmentation	3–6
Smith [35], 2003	20% solution, 2 sessions	Face, scalp	1	35	Blue light (417) or PDL (595)	80% CR for AKs with blue light; 60% CR for PDL; both demonstrated improvement in global photodamage, tactile roughness, hyperpigmentation	1
Touma [12], 2004	20% solution	Facial AKs and mild-moderate photodamage	1–3	17	Blue light (417)	Improvement in photodamage markers, including skin quality, fine rhytides, sallowness	1–5
Avram [61], 2004	20% solution	Facial photodamage (with AKs) treated with 1 ALA-IPL session	1	17	IPL	69% CR of AKs; improvement in telangiectasias, dyspigmentation, skin texture	3
Alster [62], 2005	20% solution	Split-face comparison, IPL vs. ALA-IPL	1–3	10	IPL (500–1,200)	ALA-IPL-treated side showed greater improvement	6
Dover [63], 2005	20% solution	Split-face comparison, IPL vs. ALA-IPL (5 treatment sessions)	0.5–1	20	IPL (515–1,200)	Greater improvement in ALA-IPL over IPL only for global photoaging, pigmentation, and fine lines only	1

Table 3. Continued

First author, year	ALA preparation	Location of photodamage/ study design	Incubation period, h	Patients, n	Light source (emission λ, nm)	Response	Follow-up, months
Key [67], 2005	20% solution	Face, subpurpuric doses of PDL	1	12	PDL (585)	Improvement in majority of photodamage parameters with ALA-PDL; no improvement with PDL alone	1
Lowe [72], 2005	5–20% cream	Forearm, periorbital	0.5–2	6	Red light (633)	Mild improvement noted in photoaging	0.25
Marmur [64], 2005	20% solution	Split-face comparison, IPL vs. ALA-IPL (1 treatment)	1	7	IPL	Microscopic changes demonstrated greater type I collagen on ALA-IPL side	N/A
Gold [89], 2006	20% solution	Split-face comparison, IPL vs. ALA-IPL (3 treatment sessions)	0.5–1	16	IPL (550/570 cutoff filters 1,200)	ALA-IPL results superior to IPL alone	1–3
Serrano [90], 2009	1–2% gel	Multiple application, low-concentration ALA-PDT to face, neck, hands (3 treatment sessions)	0.5–1	8/26 patients with photo-aging; 18/26treated for acne, vitiligo	IPL (530–1,200) or yellow-red lamp (550–630)	90% of cases with hyperpigmentation improvement; erythema (85%), skin texture (100%)	6
Park [59], 2010	20% cream	Two ALA-PDT at 1-month interval, repeated (2 sessions) after 1 month if required	4	14 with 1–3 AKs on the face and photo-damage	Red light (580–740 nm), dose of 100 J/cm^2, 100 mW/cm^2	82.6% CR of AKs 1 month after last treatment, microscopic analysis showed increased expression of type I and III procollagen, reduced elastotic material, decreased levels of MMP 1, 3, and 12	1 month after last treatment

Table 3. Continued

First author, year	ALA preparation	Location of photodamage/ study design	Incubation period, h	Patients, n	Light source (emission λ, nm)	Response	Follow-up, months
Clementoni [68], 2010	20% solution	Face, pretreatment with a microneedle roller followed by ALA-PDT	1	21	IPL (560 nm, cutoff filter 1,200) and red LED light (630 nm)	Improvement in photodamage markers, including fine lines, mottled pigmentation, sallowness, tactile roughness, telangiectasias	6
Xi [91], 2011	5 and 10% cream	Face, split-face comparison, IPL vs. ALA-IPL (3 treatment sessions) in Chinese patients	1	26	IPL (560 and 590, cutoff filter 1,200 nm)	Greater improvement in global score for photoaging, fine lines, coarse wrinkles; PIH was higher on the ALA-IPL PDT side (22 vs. 15% on the IPL-only side)	2
Piccioni [65], 2011	0.5% liposomal spray	Periorbital and nasolabial fold wrinkles	1	30	IPL (590–1,200)	Both areas showed statistical improvement in fine lines; improvement was greater for periorbital lines than for nasolabial folds; 47% of subjects graded their improvement as significant	3

CR = Complete response; MMP = matrix metalloproteinase; PIH = postinflammatory hyperpigmentation.

decreased after treatment as well as the expression of matrix metalloproteinases 1, 3, and 12. Collectively, these histological changes indicated restoration of photoaged skin with ALA-PDT.

Intense Pulsed Light

IPL treatments improve many of the signs of photoaging, including pigmentation in the form of solar lentigines, erythema, and telangiectasias due to vascular ectasia/damage, as well as fine wrinkling [39]. Like the PDL, IPL treatments also promote neocollagenesis [60]. Although IPL alone has been proven effective in the treatment of photodamage, the addition of ALA to IPL treatment appears to be more effective in treating photodamaged skin. Clinical examples of ALA-IPL treatment for photorejuvenation are illustrated in figures 4 and 6.

In 2002, Ruiz-Rodriguez et al. [56] investigated the treatment of photodamage and AKs using two treatments of ALA-PDT with IPL as the light source for photorejuvenation spaced 1 month apart. Treatments were well tolerated. At the 3-month follow-up, 87% of AKs were cleared, and marked cosmetic improvement was noted in wrinkling, coarse skin texture, pigmentary changes, and telangiectasias. Avram and Goldman [61] evaluated the combined use of ALA-IPL for the treatment of photorejuvenation and AKs with one treatment session. Sixty-nine percent of the AKs responded to the use of ALA-IPL. Patients displayed a 69% AK clearance rate, a 55% improvement in telangiectasias, 48% improvement in pigment irregularities, and 25% improvement in skin texture.

Alster et al. [62] also examined the use of IPL in ALA-PDT. Clinical improvement scores were noted to be higher on the side of the face treated with the combination of ALA IPL. They concluded that the combination of topical ALA with IPL is safe and more effective than IPL alone for the treatment of facial rejuvenation. A similar split-face study by Dover et al. [63] treated 20 subjects with three split-face treatments 3 weeks apart. They concluded ALA-IPL resulted in greater improvement in global photoaging (80 vs. 50%) and mottled pigmentation (95 vs. 65%). Successful results were also noted for fine lines for the ALA-IPL side compared to the IPL side alone (55 vs. 20%). Although tactile roughness and sallowness were noticeably better, pretreatment with ALA did not enhance the results of using IPL alone. Marmur et al. [64] demonstrated a greater increase in type I collagen in the subjects receiving ALA-IPL as opposed to IPL alone.

The effect of fine line reduction using IPL combined with a novel 0.5% 5-aminolevulinic liposomal spray was investigated by Piccioni et al. [65]. Thirty subjects received three treatments every 3 weeks, and improvements in the appearance of periorbital and nasolabial wrinkles were evaluated using a modified Fitzpatrick Wrinkle Scale. Three months after the final treatment, significant reduction in fine lines was seen in both treatment areas; however, a greater improvement was noted in the periorbital areas. Subject satisfaction was high, with overall improvement rated as excellent in 47% of subjects.

The effects of increasing IPL fluence on AK lesion clearance and cosmesis was investigated by Haddad et al. [66]. Twenty-four subjects were randomized to receive a single treatment with one of five regimens: IPL alone, or ALA-PDT with IPL using fluences of 20, 25, 40, or 50 J/cm^2. The study found that lesion counts gradually decreased with progressive increases in fluence (56% with 50 J/cm^2, 50% with 40 J/cm^2, 32% in 25 J/cm^2, 20% in 20 J/cm^2, and 7% with IPL alone); however, the improvement in photorejuvenation was not different between the five groups.

Yellow-Orange Light – Pulsed Dye Laser
PDLs have also been studied as a light source for photorejuvenation in ALA-PDT. PDL targets oxyhemoglobin as a chromophore according to the theory of selective photothermolysis. But thermal energy generated in the surrounding areas adjacent to targeted blood vessels may also result in photorejuvenative effects. Subpurpuric doses from the PDL alter dermal collagen and may improve skin texture [39]. Alexiades-Armenakas and Geronemus [29] found ALA-PDT with the 595-nm PDL was successful in treating face and scalp AKs and photorejuvenation. Key [67] treated 14 patients with long-incubation ALA (12 h) followed by photoactivation using PDL. Improvement was noted following ALA-PDL in terms of skin texture, tactile quality, and brown spots, although the degree of vascularity and seborrheic keratoses were unaffected by treatment. The lack of improvement in blood vessel lesions in this study is curious given that PDL targets the vasculature.

Combination Therapy with Aminolevulinic Acid and Photodynamic Therapy
A combination of a microneedling roller (108 μm in width and 300 μm in depth) prior to ALA incubation (1 h) in order to maximize epidermal penetration followed by irradiation with both red light (630 nm) and broadband pulsed light in a single treatment has been studied in 21 patients by Clementoni et al. [68]. Six months after treatment, 76.2% scored themselves an overall improvement >75%, and statistically significant improvement was observed in the global photoaging scores, fine lines, mottled pigmentation, sallowness, tactile roughness, and telangiectasias 3 months after treatment.

Enhanced efficacy of PDT after fractional resurfacing was observed by Ruiz-Rodríguez et al. [69] in 4 patients treated in the perioral area. First the 1,550-nm fractional nonablative laser was applied periorally, immediately followed by MAL-PDT (3-hour occlusion, illumination with red LED 634 nm, 37 J/cm^2) on half of the perioral area. Two treatment sessions were administered 3 weeks apart. Twelve weeks after the last treatment, a blinded investigator found increased improvement in superficial wrinkles in 3 of 4 patients on the combined treatment side as compared to the 1,550-nm fractional laser alone. The 1,550-nm nonablative fractional laser has also been used to enhance drug delivery with ALA. The authors found enhanced ALA penetration with increasing fluence of the nonablative fractionated laser [70].

Clinical Technique and Treatment Protocol

For photorejuvenation, we use the identical protocol as the one we have previously described for AK treatment (table 2). We counsel our patients to expect three to four sessions of PDT when treating photorejuvenation, especially when sebaceous hyperplasia is present. These recommendations are consistent with the recommendations of the American Society of Photodynamic Therapy [13].

Practical Considerations in Photodynamic Therapy

Exclusion Criteria

Patients should be screened for important exclusion criteria prior to undergoing PDT. A history of photosensitivity including porphyria, photodermatoses, and photosensitizing medication use should preclude treatment [28, 57, 71]. Many studies have excluded patients from treatment if they have undergone treatment with systemic retinoids, chemotherapeutic agents, or immunotherapy in the past 6 months [20, 71, 72]. Pregnant or nursing women and individuals with an active infection should not undergo treatment [22, 73]. Jeffes et al. [71] recommended patients refrain from topical retinoids, α-hydroxy acids, and chemical peels approximately 1 month prior to treatment.

Side Effects and Management of Complications

Some mild adverse events following PDT are expected and the result of the phototoxic nature of treatment. Pain and burning may be experienced during light irradiation. The precise mechanism of pain is not fully elucidated but likely involves nerve stimulation and/or tissue damage [74]. Shorter incubation times decrease the severity of side effects. Expected phototoxic side effects include erythema, edema, stinging/burning, pruritus, and crusting. Pigmentary changes, whealing, and vesiculation may also occur [18, 23, 73, 75]. Erythema and mild crusting occur in most patients following treatment, usually resolving in 1–2 weeks (fig. 7) [38]. Hypopigmentation is rare, and hyperpigmentation, with an incidence as high as 27% following ALA-PDT [73], is usually mild in nature. More pronounced reactions are correlated with disease burden. Typically, repeat treatments are less painful than previous ones.

In patients with extensive phototoxic reactions, especially in cases when patients are exposed to UV radiation in the 24–36 h following treatment, topical therapy may be necessary to address erythema, edema, and crusting. Topical steroid creams and ice packs may be used on the treated area until the symptoms subside. All patients should be screened for a history of cold sores and appropriate herpes simplex virus prophylaxis begun prior to treatment in such cases [6].

Pain management, especially with shorter incubation times (e.g. 1 h), is usually a nonissue. Reassurance to the patient and 'talk-esthesia' by a caring member of the clinical staff is usually more than adequate to comfort any patient anxiety and pain. However, the use of cooling fans, Avene Thermal Water Spray, forced air cooling systems, Xylocaine spray, and even oral nonnarcotic pain medication have been used successfully to mitigate pain during ALA-PDT [12, 38, 73].

A review study by Warren et al. [74] of 43 articles consisting of clinical PDT trials (2000–2008) that used ALA or MAL was performed to summarize the effectiveness of interventions to reduce PDT-related pain and to explore contributing factors to pain induction. Their consensus opinion is that, in general, topical anesthetics do not work, and cooling the skin with either ice water or with a high-airflow cooling device (such as Zimmer MedizinSystems, Irvine, Calif., USA) represents the best topical intervention to control the pain during PDT. They also found that pain intensity is associated with lesion size and location; certain diagnoses, particularly plaque-type psoriasis, appear to generate the highest PDT-related pain scores. Inconsistent results were encountered for the correlation of pain with light source, wavelength of light, fluence rate, and total light dose. Similarly, Buinauskaite et al. [76] discovered pain following ALA-PDT was more severe with AKs >130 mm [2]. Additionally, ALA-PDT of facial AKs were twice as painful as scalp AKs. PDT procedural pain is also amplified as device fluence is increased [77].

Although the use of forced airflow cooling appears to be effective in reducing pain during PDT, a recent nonrandomized retrospective observational controlled study conducted by Tyrrell et al. [78] demonstrated that patients using an airflow cooling device throughout treatment presented significantly less PpIX photobleaching than the control group, translating into decreased response rates. As demonstrated by previous studies [79, 80], the level of PpIX photobleaching correlates to cell death, and therefore tumor clearance rates, and might be the reason that utilization of airflow cooling during light irradiation lowers the potential efficacy of the treatment. It is proposed that the low temperature of air used may cause local vasoconstriction, reducing reactive oxygen species production and thus limiting clinical effectiveness.

Not unexpectedly, if patients require a second treatment, the adverse effects as well as treatment pain are usually much less than experienced with the initial treatment. We believe that the decrease is due to the resolution of most of the clinical and subclinical photodamage which occurs during the initial treatment.

Conclusion

PDT is a safe and effective treatment for nonhyperkeratotic lesions. Efficacy is reduced when treating the extremities; however, occlusion, heating pads, prolonging incubation times, and utilization of combination therapies can all help improve clearance rates in these locations. Although ALA-PDT is FDA approved for use with a blue light source, other laser and light sources have demonstrated promise in the treatment of AKs during PDT. Shorter incubation times maintain AK clearance rates but decrease the occurrence of phototoxic adverse events. With careful patient selection, PDT allows selective field treatment of precancerous skin lesions along with an improvement in overall photodamage. Patient satisfaction is high and cosmetic results can be excellent.

References

1 Kennedy JC, Pottier RH, Pross DC, et al: Photodynamic therapy with endogenous protoporphyrin IX: basic principles and present clinical experiences. J Photochem Photobiol B 1990;6:143–148.

2 Peng Q, Warloe T, Berg C, Moan J, Kongshaug M, et al: 5-Aminolevulinic acid-based photodynamic therapy: clinical research and future challenges. Cancer 1997;79:2282–2308.

3 Ko DY, Kim KH, Song KH: Comparative study of photodynamic therapy with topical methyl aminolevulinate versus 5-aminolevulinic acid for facial actinic keratosis with long-term follow-up. Ann Dermatol 2014;26:321–331.

4 Soret JL: Recherches sur l'absorption des rayons ultra-violets par diverses substances. Arch Sci Phys Nat 1883;10:430–485.

5 Calzavara-Pinton PG, Venturini M, Sala R: Photodynamic therapy: update 2006. Part 1. Photochemistry and photobiology. J Eur Acad Dermatol Venereol 2007;21:293–302.

6 Nootheti PK, Goldman MP: Aminolevulinic acid-photodynamic therapy for photorejuvenation. Dermatol Clin 2007;25:35–45.

7 Ericson MB, Sandberg C, Stenquist B, Gudmundson F, et al: Photodynamic therapy of actinic keratosis at varying fluence rates: assessment of photobleaching, pain and primary clinical outcome. Br J Dermatol 2004;151:1204–1212.

8 Nakaseko H, Kobayashi M, Akita Y, Tamada Y, et al: Histological changes and involvement of apoptosis after photodynamic therapy for actinic keratoses. Br J Dermatol 2003;148:122–127.

9 Wolf P, Rieger E, Kerl H: Topical photodynamic therapy with endogenous porphyrins after application of 5-aminolevulinic acid. J Am Acad Dermatol 1993;28:17–21.

10 MacCormack MA: Photodynamic therapy in dermatology: an update on applications and outcomes. Semin Cutan Med Surg 2008;27:52–62.

11 Product information (package insert): Levulan® Kerastick™ (aminolevulinic acid HCl) for topical solution, 20%. DUSA Pharmaceuticals, Wilmington, 2009.

12 Touma D, Yaar M, Whitehead S, Konnikov N, et al: A trial of short incubation, broad-area photodynamic therapy for facial actinic keratoses and diffuse photodamage. Arch Dermatol 2004;140:33–40.

13 Nestor MS, Gold MH, Kauvar ANB, Taub AF, et al: The use of photodynamic therapy in dermatology: results of a consensus conference. J Drugs Dermatol 2006;5:140–154.

14 Goldberg DJ: Photodynamic therapy in skin rejuvenation. Clin Dermatol 2008;26:608–613.

15 Nakano A, Tamada Y, Watanabe D, Ishida N, et al: A pilot study to assess the efficacy of photodynamic therapy for Japanese patients with actinic keratosis in relation to lesion size and histological severity. Photodermatol Photoimmunol Photomed 2009;25:37–40.

16 Peng Q, Warloe T, Berg K, Moan J, et al: 5-Aminolevulinic acid-based photodynamic therapy. Cancer 1997;79:2282–2308.

17 Zakhary K, Ellis DAF: Applications of aminolevulinic acid-based photodynamic therapy in cosmetic facial plastic practices. Facial Plast Surg 2005;21:110–116.

18 Kalka K, Merk H, Mukhtar H: Photodynamic therapy in dermatology. J Am Acad Dermatol 2000;42:389–413.

19 Clark C, Bryden A, Dawe R, Moseley H, et al: Topical 5-aminolevulinic acid photodynamic therapy for cutaneous lesions: outcome and comparison of light sources. Photodermatol Photoimmunol Photomed 2003;19:134–141.

20 Kalisiak MS, Rao J: Photodynamic therapy for actinic keratoses. Dermatol Clin 2007;25:15–23.

21 Glogau RG: The risk of progression to invasive disease. J Am Acad Dermatol 2000;42(1 pt 2):23–24.

22 Jeffes EW, McCullough JL, Weinstein GD, Kaplan R, Glazer SD, Taylor JR: Photodynamic therapy of actinic keratoses with topical aminolevulinic acid hydrochloride and fluorescent blue light. J Am Acad Dermatol 2001;45:96–104.

23 Szeimies RM, Karrer S, Radakovic-Fijan S, et al: Photodynamic therapy using topical methyl 5-aminolevulinate compared with cryotherapy for actinic keratosis: a prospective, randomized study. J Am Acad Dermatol 2002;47:258–262.

24 Gold MH: Pharmacoeconomic analysis of the treatment of multiple actinic keratoses. J Drugs Dermatol 2008;7:23–25.
25 Kurwa HA, Yong-Gee SA, Seed PT, et al: A randomized paired comparison of photodynamic therapy and topical 5-fluorouracil in the treatment of actinic keratoses. J Am Acad Dermatol 1999;41:414–418.
26 Gupta AK, Paquet M: Network meta-analysis of the outcome 'participant complete clearance' in nonimmunosuppressed participants of eight interventions for actinic keratosis: a follow-up on a Cochrane review. Br J Dermatol 2013;169:250–259.
27 Tierney EP, Eide MJ, Jacobsen, Ozog D: Photodynamic therapy for actinic keratoses: survey of patient perceptions of treatment satisfaction and outcomes. J Cosmet Laser Ther 2008;10:81–86.
28 Goldman MP, Atkin DH: ALA/PDT in the treatment of actinic keratosis: spot versus confluent therapy. J Cosmet Laser Ther 2003;5:107–110.
29 Alexiades-Armenakas MR, Geronemus RG: Laser-mediated photodynamic therapy of actinic keratoses. Arch Dermatol 2003;139;1313–1320.
30 Ross EV, Anderson RR: Laser-tissue interactions; in Goldman MP (ed): Cutaneous and Cosmetic Laser Surgery. Philadelphia, Elsevier, 2006, pp 1–26.
31 Ormrod D, Jarvis B: Topical aminolevulinic acid HCl photodynamic therapy. Am J Clin Dermatol 2000;2:133–139.
32 Piacquadio DJ, Chen DM, Farber HF, et al: Photodynamic therapy with aminolevulinic acid topical solution and visible blue light in the treatment of multiple actinic keratoses of the face and scalp: investigator-blinded, phase 3, multicenter trials. Arch Dermatol 2004;140:41–46.
33 Taub AF, Garretson CB: A randomized, blinded, bilateral intraindividual, vehicle-controlled trial of the use of photodynamic therapy with 5-aminolevulinic acid and blue light for the treatment of actinic keratosis of the upper extremities. J Drugs Dermatol 2011;10:1049–1056.
34 Schmieder GJ, Huang EY, Jarratt M: A multicenter, randomized, vehicle-controlled phase 2 study of blue light photodynamic therapy with aminolevulinic acid HCl 20% topical solution for the treatment of actinic keratoses on the upper extremities: the effect of occlusion during the drug incubation period. J Drugs Dermatol 2012;11:1483–1489.
35 Smith S, Piacquadio D, Morhenn V, Atkin D: Short incubation PDT versus 5-FU in treating actinic keratoses. J Drugs Dermatol 2003;2:629–635.
36 Itoh Y, Nineomiya Y, Henta T, Tajima S, et al: Topical delta-aminolevulinic acid-based photodynamic therapy for Japanese actinic keratoses. J Dermatol 2000;27:513–518.
37 Varma S, Wilson H, Kurwa HA, Gambles B, et al: Bowen's disease, solar keratoses and superficial basal cell carcinomas treated by photodynamic therapy using a large-field incoherent light source. Br J Dermatol 2001;144:567–574.
38 Moseley H, Ibbotson S, Woods J, Brancaleon L, Lesar A, Goodman C, Ferguson J: Clinical and research applications of photodynamic therapy in dermatology: experience of the Scottish PDT centre. Lasers Surg Med 2006;38:403–416.
39 DeHoratius DM, Dover JS: Nonablative tissue remodeling and photorejuvenation. Clin Dermatol 2007;25:474–479.
40 Kim HS, Yoo JY, Cho KH, Kwon OS, et al: Topical photodynamic therapy using intense pulsed light for treatment of actinic keratosis: clinical and histopathologic evaluation. Dermatol Surg 2005;31:33–37.
41 Gilbert D: Treatment of actinic keratoses with sequential combination of 5-fluorouracil and photodynamic therapy. J Drugs Dermatol 2005;4:161–163.
42 Martin G: Prospective, case-based assessment of sequential therapy with topical fluorouracil cream 0.5% and ALA-PDT for the treatment of actinic keratosis. J Drugs Dermatol 2011;10:372–378.
43 Shaffelburg M: Treatment of actinic keratoses with sequential use of photodynamic therapy and imiquimod 5% cream. J Drugs Dermatol 2009;8:35–39.
44 Tanaka N, Ohata C, Ishii N, et al: Comparative study for the effect of photodynamic therapy, imiquimod immunotherapy and combination of both therapies on 40 lesions of actinic keratosis in Japanese patients. J Dermatol 2013;40:962–967.
45 Jang YH, Lee DJ, Shin J, et al: Photodynamic therapy with ablative carbon dioxide fractional laser in treatment of actinic keratosis. Ann Dermatol 2013;25: 417–422.
46 Markham T, Collins P: Topical 5-aminolaevulinic acid photodynamic therapy for extensive scalp actinic keratoses. Br J Dermatol 2001;145:502–504.
47 Uebelhoer NS, Dover J: Photodynamic therapy for cosmetic applications. Dermatol Ther 2005;18:242–252.
48 Lee WR, Tsai RY, Fang CL, Liu CJ, Hu CH, Fang JY: Microdermabrasion as a novel tool to enhance drug delivery via the skin: an animal study. Dermatol Surg 2006;32:1013–1022.
49 Katz BE, Truong S, Maiwald DC, Frew KE, George BA: Efficacy of microdermabrasion preceding ALA application in reducing the incubation time of ALA in laser PDT. J Drugs Dermatol 2007;6:140–142.
50 Gollnick SO, Liu X, Owczarczak B, Musser DA, Henderson BW: Altered expression of interleukin 6 and interleukin 10 as a result of photodynamic therapy in vivo. Cancer Res 1997;57:3904–3909.

51 Borelli C, Herzinger T, Merk K, Berking C, Kunte C, Plewig G, Degitz K: Effect of subcutaneous infiltration anesthesia on pain in photodynamic therapy: a controlled open pilot trial. Dermatol Surg 2007;33: 314–318.

52 Willey A, Anderson RR, Sakamoto FH: Temperature-modulated photodynamic therapy for the treatment of actinic keratosis on the extremities: a pilot study. Dermatol Surg 2014;40:1094–1102.

53 Oseroff A: PDT as a cytotoxic agent and biological response modifier: implications for cancer prevention and treatment in immunosuppressed and immunocompetent patients. J Invest Dermatol 2006; 126:542–544.

54 Dragieva G, Hafner J, Dummer R, Schmid-Grendelmeier P, et al: Topical photodynamic therapy in the treatment of actinic keratoses and Bowen's disease in transplant recipients. Transplantation 2004;17:115–121.

55 de Graaf YGL, Kennedy C, Wolterbeek R, Collen AFS, et al: Photodynamic therapy does not prevent cutaneous squamous-cell carcinoma in organ-transplant recipients: results of a randomized-controlled trial. J Invest Dermatol 2006;126:569–574.

56 Ruiz-Rodriguez R, Sanz-Sánchez T, Córdoba S: Photodynamic photorejuvenation. Dermatol Surg 2002; 28:742–744.

57 Zane C, Capezzera R, Sala R, Venturini M, Calzavara-Pinton P: Clinical and echographic analysis of photodynamic therapy using methylaminolevulinate as sensitizer in the treatment of photodamaged facial skin. Lasers Surg Med 2007;39:203–209.

58 Jeffes EWB: Levulan: the first approved topical photosensitizer for the treatment of actinic keratosis. J Dermatol Treat 2002;13:S19–S23.

59 Park MY, Sohn S, Lee E, Kim YC: Photorejuvenation induced by 5-aminolevulinic acid photodynamic therapy in patients with actinic keratosis: a histologic analysis. J Am Acad Dermatol 2010;62:85–95.

60 Goldberg DJ: New collagen formation after dermal remodeling with intense pulsed light sources. J Cutan Laser Ther 2000;2:59–61.

61 Avram DK, Goldman MP: Effectiveness and safety of ALA-IPL in treating actinic keratoses and photodamage. J Drugs Dermatol 2004;3:S36–S39.

62 Alster TS, Tanzi EL, Welch EC: Photorejuvenation of facial skin with topical 20% 5-aminolevulinic acid and intense pulsed light treatment: a split-face comparison study. J Drugs Dermatol 2005;4:35–38.

63 Dover JS, Bhatia AC, Stewart B, Arndt KA: Topical 5-aminolevulinic acid combined with intense pulsed light in the treatment of photoaging. Arch Dermatol 2005;141:1247–1252.

64 Marmur ES, Phelps R, Goldberg DJ: Ultrastructural changes seen after ALA-IPL photorejuvenation: a pilot study. J Cosmet Laser Ther 2005;7:21–44.

65 Piccioni A, Fargnoli MC, Schoinas S, et al: Efficacy and tolerability of 5-aminolevulinic acid 0.5% liposomal spray and intense pulsed light in wrinkle reduction of photodamaged skin. J Dermatol Treat 2011;22:247–253.

66 Haddad A, Santos ID, Gragnsni A, et al: The effect of increasing fluence rates on the treatment of actinic keratosis and photodamage by photodynamic therapy with 5-aminolevulinic acid and intense pulsed light. Photomed Laser Surg 2011;29:427–432.

67 Key DJ: Aminolevulinic acid-pulsed dye laser photodynamic therapy for the treatment of photoaging. Cosmet Dermatol 2005;18:31–36.

68 Clementoni MT, Roscher MB, Munavalli GS: Photodynamic photorejuvenation of the face with a combination of microneedling, red light, and broadband pulsed light. Lasers Surg Med 2010;42:150–159.

69 Ruiz-Rodriguez R, López L, Candelas D, Zelickson B: Enhanced efficacy of photodynamic therapy after fractional resurfacing: fractional photodynamic rejuvenation. J Drugs Dermatol 2007;6:818–820.

70 Lim HK, Jeong KH, Kim NI, et al: Nonablative fractional laser as a tool to facilitate skin penetration of 5-aminolaevulinic acid with minimal skin disruption: a preliminary study. Br J Dermatol 2014;170: 1336–1340.

71 Jeffes WJ, McCullagh JL, Weinstein GD, Fergin PE, et al: Photodynamic therapy of actinic keratosis with topical 5-aminolaevulinic acid. Arch Dermatol 1997; 133:727–732.

72 Lowe NJ, Lowe P: Pilot study to determine the efficacy of ALA-PDT photorejuvenation for the treatment of facial ageing. J Cosmet Laser Ther 2005;7: 159–162.

73 Tschen EH, Wong DS, Pariser DM, Dunlap FE, Houlihan A, Ferdon MB: Photodynamic therapy using aminolaevulinic acid for patients with nonhyperkeratotic actinic keratoses of the face and scalp: phase IV mulicentre clinical trial with 12-month follow up. Br J Dermatol 2006;155:1262–1269.

74 Warren CB, Karai LJ, Vidimos A, Maytin EV: Pain associated with aminolevulinic acid-photodynamic therapy of skin disease. J Am Acad Dermatol 2009; 61:1033–1043.

75 Gholam P, Kroehl V, Enk AH: Dermatology life quality index and side effects after topical photodynamic therapy of actinic keratosis. Dermatology 2013;223:253–259.

76 Buinauskaite E, Zalinkevicius R, Buinauskaite J, et al: Pain during topical photodynamic therapy of actinic keratoses with 5-aminolevulinic acid and red light source: randomized controlled trial. Photodermatol Photoimmunol Photomed 2013;29:173–181.

77 Apalla Z, Sotiriou E, Panagiotidou D, et al: The impact of different fluence rates on pain and clinical outcome in patients with actinic keratoses treated with photodynamic therapy. Photodermatol Photoimmunol Photomed 2011;27:181–185.
78 Tyrrell J, Campbell SM, Curnow A: The effect of air cooling pain relief on protoporphyrin IX photobleaching and clinical efficacy during dermatological photodynamic therapy. J Photochem Photobiol B 2011;103:1–7.
79 Tyrrell J, Campbell SM, Curnow A: The relationship between protoporphyrin IX photobleaching during real-time dermatological methyl-aminoluvinate photodynamic therapy (MAL-PDT) and subsequent clinical outcome. Lasers Surg Med 2010;42:613–619.
80 Ascencio M, Collinet P, Farine MO, Mordon S: Protoporphyrin IX fluorescence photobleaching is a useful tool to predict the response of rat ovarian cancer following hexaminolevulinate photodynamic therapy. Lasers Surg Med 2008;40:332–341.
81 Morton CA, Whitehurst C, Moseley H, et al: Development of an alternative light source to lasers for photodynamic therapy: clinical evaluation in the treatment of pre-malignant non-melanoma skin cancer. Lasers Med Sci 1995;10:165–171.
82 Fijan S, Honigsmann H, Ortel B: Photodynamic therapy of epithelial skin tumors with delta-aminolaevulinic acid and desferrioxamine. Br J Dermatol 1995;133:282–288.
83 Szeimies RM, Karrer S, Sauerwald A, Landthaler M: Photodynamic therapy with topical application of 5-aminolevulinic acid in the treatment of actinic keratoses: an initial clinical study. Dermatology 1996; 192:246–251.
84 Fink-Puches R, Hofer A, Smolle J, Kerl H, et al: Primary clinical response and long-term follow-up of solar keratoses treated with topically applied 5-aminolevulinic acid and irradiation by different wave bands of light. J Photochem Photobiol 1997;41:145–151.
85 Fritsch C, Stege H, Saalmann G, Goerz G, et al: Green light is effective and less painful than red light in photodynamic therapy of facial solar keratoses. Photodermatol Photoimmunol Photomed 1997;13:181–185.
86 Karrer S, Bäumler W, Abels C, Hohenleutner U, et al: Long-pulse dye laser for photodynamic therapy: investigations in vitro and in vivo. Lasers Surg Med 1999;25:51–59.
87 Dijkstra AT, Majoie IML, van Dongen JWF, van Weelden H, et al: Photodynamic therapy with violet light and topical δ-aminolaevulinic acid in the treatment of actinic keratosis, Bowen's disease and basal cell carcinoma. J Eur Acad Dermatol Venereol 2001; 15:550–554.
88 Cai H, Wang YX, Sun P, et al: Photodynamic therapy for facial actinic keratosis: a clinical and histological study in Chinese patients. Photodiagnosis Photodyn Ther 2013;10:260–265.
89 Gold MH, Bradshaw VL, Boring MM, Bridges TM, et al: Split-face comparison of photodynamic therapy with 5-aminolevulinic acid and intense pulsed light versus intense pulsed light alone for photodamage. Dermatol Surg 2006;32:795–803.
90 Serrano G, Lorente M, Reyes M, Millán F, et al: Photodynamic therapy with low-strength ALA, repeated applications and short contact periods (40–60 min) in acne, photoaging, and vitiligo. J Drugs Dermatol 2009;8:562–568.
91 Xi Z, Shuxian Y, Zhong L, Hui Q, Yan W, et al: Topical 5-aminolevulinic acid with intense pulsed light versus intense pulsed light for photodamage in Chinese patients. Dermatol Surg 2011;37:31–40.

Jennifer D. Peterson, MD
Suzanne Bruce and Associates
23510 Kingsland Boulevard, Suite 300
Katy, TX 77494 (USA)
E-Mail Jenniferpetersonmd@gmail.com

Gold MH (ed): Cosmetic Photodynamic Therapy. Aesthet Dermatol. Basel, Karger, 2016, vol 3, pp 36–63
DOI: 10.1159/000441510

Topical Methyl Aminolevulinate-Photodynamic Therapy for the Treatment of Actinic Keratoses and Photorejuvenation

Peter Foley

Department of Medicine (Dermatology), St. Vincent's Hospital Melbourne, University of Melbourne, Fitzroy, Vic., and Department of Dermatology, Skin and Cancer Foundation, Carlton, Vic., Australia

Abstract

Background: Fair-skinned individuals exposed to ultraviolet radiation in sunlight age prematurely (photoaging) and develop actinic (solar) keratoses (AKs). Photoaging is characterized by fine lines, wrinkles, uneven or mottled pigmentation, sallow complexion, tactile roughness, erythema, and telangiectasia. The risk of malignant transformation of AKs is still debated, but as there is as yet no means to distinguish those that will transform or progress and those that will not, the ILDS (International League of Dermatological Societies) guidelines recommend adequate treatment. Methyl aminolevulinate (MAL) photodynamic therapy (PDT) is now an established treatment for AKs that has proven efficacy and resulted in excellent cosmetic outcomes. Not only the absence of scarring or pigment changes after PDT, but also the coincidental improvement in signs of skin aging, has prompted a closer examination of the aesthetic benefits/effects (and the characterization of the mode of action) in specific targeted clinical studies. In addition, a major approved variation in MAL-PDT has been the introduction of daylight PDT utilizing visible wavelengths in sunlight to activate the protoporphyrins produced intracellularly in response to MAL exposure. The objective of this chapter is to report the efficacy of topical MAL-PDT for AK, its cosmetic outcomes and side effects. Multiple electronic databases were searched for studies involving MAL-PDT, AK, and photoaging. The Cochrane Central Register of Controlled Trials was also searched. Additionally, cited references of all trials identified and key review articles were assessed. A total of 18 studies which studied MAL-PDT to treat AKs were included in this review. Four studies compared MAL-PDT and cryotherapy; 3 other studies compared MAL-PDT with placebo cream. Only 1 study compared MAL-PDT with both cryotherapy and placebo, while 1 report examined proprietary MAL-PDT in comparison with compounded aminolevulinic acid (ALA) PDT. Two studies compared differences in treatment regimens; dose, and treatment interval. One study compared MAL-PDT with imiquimod 5% cream, 1 with diclofenac in hyaluronic acid gel, and 2 with new ALA formulations. Three studies examined daylight MAL-PDT for AKs. MAL-PDT is effective as a treatment for AK lesions, especially on the face and scalp. The cosmetic outcome is excellent and superior to cryotherapy in terms of minimum skin discoloration and scarring. The side effects, including skin 'burning', pain, and erythema, have been reported as tolerable. The introduction of daylight MAL-PDT has removed pain, a potential barrier to utilization of the procedure, from the decision-making process. Further work is required to explore the application of MAL-PDT as a photorejuvenation technique.

Introduction

Description of the Conditions

Disease Definition and Clinical Features

Fair-skinned individuals exposed to ultraviolet (UV) radiation in sunlight age prematurely (photoaging) and develop actinic (solar) keratoses (AKs). Photoaging is characterized by fine lines, wrinkles, uneven or mottled pigmentation, sallow complexion, tactile roughness, erythema, and telangiectasia.

Methyl aminolevulinate (MAL) photodynamic therapy (PDT) is now an established treatment for AKs that has proven efficacy and shown excellent cosmetic outcomes. Not only the absence of scarring or pigment changes after PDT, but also the coincidental improvement in signs of skin aging, has prompted a closer examination of the aesthetic benefits/effects (and the characterization of the mode of action) in specific targeted clinical studies. The published regimes employed in examining the photorejuvenation effects of PDT deviate considerably from those licensed for treatment of AK. In addition, a major approved variation in MAL-PDT has been the introduction of daylight PDT utilizing visible wavelengths in sunlight to activate the protoporphyrins produced intracellularly in response to exposure to MAL.

The lesions variously referred to as AK or solar keratosis are UV radiation-induced cutaneous premalignant lesions typically seen on sun-exposed areas of skin, including the face, scalp, forearms, and dorsal hands of fair-skinned individuals. The risk of malignant transformation is still debated, but as there is as yet no means to distinguish those that will transform/progress and those that will not, the ILDS (International League of Dermatological Societies) guidelines recommend adequate treatment [1].

Clinically, or macroscopically, AK presents as erythematous keratotic patches/macules, papules, or plaques. Most are slowly growing pink, red, or brown lesions with nonflaking scale. AK may become hypertrophic/thickened or hyperkeratotic/horny, and on occasion bleed. Most AK lesions are asymptomatic but can exhibit symptoms such as burning, stinging, pruritus, or tenderness. AKs may occur as solitary lesions, but more commonly are multiple, and represent field changes or cancerization.

Natural History

Any individual AK may follow one of three paths: it may regress, it may persist unchanged, or it may progress to invasive squamous cell carcinoma (SCC) [2–4]. Marks et al. [5] reported that the presence of AKs is highly associated with an increased frequency of both SCC and basal cell carcinoma (BCC). Glogau [6] estimated that the rate at which an individual AK lesion may progress to SCC varies from 0.025 to 16% per year. The nature of its potential progression highlights the importance of effective therapy to eradicate the lesion.

Epidemiology and Causes

Evidence suggests that UV light by itself is sufficient to induce AK [7, 8]. Some individuals are more susceptible to develop AK: fair-skinned, fair-haired patients, who tan poorly and burn easily, often develop the lesions. In addition, UVB-specific p53 mutations, which have been demonstrated in AK, strengthen the evidence of a role for sunlight [9]. AK occurs most frequently in the elderly, especially men, who are also at highest risk for death from SCC. There is a high prevalence in immunosuppressed individuals such as organ transplant recipients and HIV patients [10]. Other possible contributory risk factors are cutaneous human papilloma virus, exposure to arsenic, and chronic sun bed use. However, AK only occurs in people who are exposed to sun [9].

Description of Interventions

Photodynamic Therapy with Methyl Aminolevulinate

MAL (Metvix™ in Australia and European countries, Metvixia in North America) is a topically applied photosensitizing precursor used to treat precancerous lesions, such as AK, and nonmelanoma skin cancer, such as superficial and nodular BCC and Bowen's disease [11]. In the United States and Canada, 5-aminolevulinic acid (ALA; Levulan™) is widely used. Evidence suggests that there is greater selectivity for neoplastic tissue with MAL in comparison to ALA [12, 13].

PDT combines the simultaneous presence of photosensitizer; in this case MAL metabolite(s), activated by an appropriate wavelength of light, in the presence of oxygen, induce intracellular damage to the target cell. Braathen et al. [14] reported in the international guidelines on the use of PDT for nonmelanoma cancer that it is important to choose an appropriate light for PDT to ensure optimal photosensitizer excitation and tissue penetration.

The Mechanism of Photodynamic Therapy with Methyl Aminolevulinate and Patient Preparation

Before MAL cream application, any crust or scales overlying lesions are gently removed to allow better skin penetration. After topical application of MAL, sufficient time, usually approximately 3 h (under occlusion, e.g. Tegaderm), is allowed to permit penetration of the active agent into the neoplastic cells, with subsequent porphyrin production and accumulation, before activation with light. During light illumination (until recently, conventionally with the Aktilite, 37 J/cm^2), photoactive porphyrins are excited to a higher energy state (triplet state). Upon returning to the resting state, this energy is transferred to oxygen molecules present, which are transformed into cytotoxic free radicals (including hydroxyl radicals) and singlet oxygen species. The target cell is destroyed by apoptosis and necrosis [15, 16]. PDT is usually well tolerated, has excellent cosmetic results, and studies have documented cure rates between 69 and 93% [17, 18]. Potential adverse effects such as initial erythema; edema; a burning sensation; pain, and crusting followed by hypo- or hyperpigmentation; ulceration, or scaling have been reported [17, 18].

The ideal treatment of AK must fulfill three criteria: it must be effective, well tolerated and have an excellent cosmetic outcome. Areas such as the face are cosmetically sensitive areas, and patients often consider this factor when choosing a treatment. MAL-PDT may be suggested as a first-line treatment for AK lesions as it is an effective and selective targeted treatment that only destroys target cells. However, to develop treatment recommendations requires sufficient evidence from clinical trials and studies. This chapter examines the efficacy, cosmetic outcomes, and side effects of MAL-PDT in comparison to placebo cream, cryotherapy, imiquimod, diclofenac [19], and ALA-PDT [20]. Previous studies have shown that MAL-PDT provides good clinical outcomes in the treatment of AK. MAL, the methyl ester of ALA, may offer an advantage over ALA in terms of deeper skin penetration [13]. Cryotherapy, though it has almost similar efficacy with MAL-PDT, is reported to have poorer cosmetic outcomes.

Method

Criteria for Considering Studies for This Review

Type of Studies

Published randomized controlled trials and open-label trials comparing the following types of treatment were included in this review:

- MAL-PDT and cryotherapy
- MAL-PDT and placebo
- MAL-PDT and ALA-PDT
- MAL-PDT and imiquimod 5% cream
- MAL-PDT and diclofenac 3% plus hyaluronic acid gel

In addition, studies evaluating doses of PDT as well as treatment intervals were also included.

Search Method for the Identification of Studies

Electronic Searches

Literature search was carried out using MEDLINE, PubMed, and Web of Science. Another literature search was undertaken using the Cochrane Central Register of Controlled Trials (CENTRAL), with citations published between 1995 and 2015. This period was chosen because MAL-PDT has been considered a new treatment and most of the studies were carried out after 2000. Articles were obtained by using the following key words: 'photodynamic therapy', 'methyl aminolevulinate' AND 'actinic keratosis', 'photodynamic therapy (PDT)' AND 'actinic keratosis', 'daylight' AND 'photodynamic therapy', 'methyl aminolevulinate' AND 'actinic keratosis', and 'photodynamic therapy', 'methyl aminolevulinate' AND 'photorejuvenation'. Studies were limited to the English language and adult participants. Other than that, two main journals, the *British Journal of Dermatology* and the *Journal of the American Academy of Dermatology*, were accessed due to their known identification for publishing the results of MAL-PDT trials. Finally, the Cochrane database of systematic reviews was used to find other journals from the references of the studies.

Searching Other Resources

Other resources such as conference presentations and the latest guidelines on the use of PDT for nonmelanoma skin cancer by Braathen et al. [14] and daylight PDT by Morton et al. [21] were reviewed. In addition, other appropriate studies, which met the inclusion and exclusion criteria, were identified from the reference list of the included studies. Journals and books about AK and PDT were searched from the citation of the latest guidelines and other studies included in the review. All the references were scanned for appropriate extraction.

Inclusion and Exclusion Criteria of the Studies

Studies that are included in this review are those that are written in the English language. Studies contained information on the primary outcome, lesion response rates, in their results. Studies are excluded if the patients involved suffered from diseases other than AKs, such as Bowen's disease and BCC. This review is specific for AK lesions and photorejuvenation only.

Type of Participants

For MAL-PDT for AK, studies must involve adults aged at least 18 years who had one or more AK lesion and were eligible for randomization to active treatment, placebo/open or other treatment. In all participants, AK lesions should be diagnosed by a dermatologist by clinical assessment.

Type of Outcome Measures

Primary Outcomes

Lesion Response to Treatment. Lesion response is classified as either (1) complete response (CR) – defined as complete disappearance of the lesion - or (2) no CR – defined as incomplete disappearance of the lesion. Outcomes were measured by lesion count by inspection, photography, and palpation from baseline to follow-up assessments, depending on the study protocol.

Secondary Outcomes

Cosmetic Effect. Cosmetic outcomes are defined as follows [17]:

- Excellent: no scarring, atrophy, or induration, and no or slight occurrence of redness or change in pigmentation compared with adjacent skin
- Good: no scarring, atrophy, or induration, but moderate redness or change in pigmentation compared to adjacent skin
- Fair: slight-to-moderate occurrence of scarring, atrophy, or induration
- Poor: extensive occurrence of scarring, atrophy, or induration

Cosmetic outcomes were assessed by a dermatologist involved in the studies.

Other Outcomes. They included side effects, which will be discussed briefly. Side effects, which were documented by the investigator, were recorded at the end of the treatment by either interview or questionnaire.

Data Extraction

The following data were extracted from each study:

- Name of the authors and the type of the study
- The primary aims of the study
- The criteria of the population of the study

- The comparator group of the study
- The results of the study

This information extracted was recorded and is presented in the Results of this review.

Assessment of Risk of Bias in Included Studies
The assessment of risk of bias (methodological quality) included an evaluation of the following components for each study:
- Randomization procedure
- Concealment of allocation
- Intention-to-treat analysis
- Blinding
- Number of patients lost to follow-up

Results

Description of the Studies Included

Table 1 illustrates the description of the studies in the review. Out of 18 studies reviewed, 4 studies compared MAL-PDT and cryotherapy; another 3 studies compared MAL-PDT with placebo cream. One study reported the outcomes of comparison with both placebo cream and cryotherapy. Three studies discussed the difference in efficacy, cosmetic outcomes, and patient preference between MAL-PDT and ALA-PDT, 2 with new ALA formulations. The study conducted by Tarstedt et al. [18] compared treatment regimens using different doses and treatment intervals between two treatments. This study was included in this review because it has sufficient information on the outcomes investigated. Similarly, a study by Caekelbergh et al. [22] was reviewed for the same reason even though its primary aim was to investigate the cost-effectiveness between MAL-PDT and cryotherapy. One study compared MAL-PDT with imiquimod 5% cream, 1 with diclofenac in hyaluronic acid gel, and 1 study examined pretreatment with nonablative fractional laser. Three studies examined daylight MAL-PDT for AK.

Methodological Quality

Table 2 describes the methodological quality of all studies included in this review. Six criteria were used to access methodological quality of the studies chosen. From table 2, all the studies had allocation concealment and intention-to-treat analysis. Studies comparing MAL-PDT with placebo and ALA-PDT, as well as those comparing the treatment regimens, were considered as good quality studies because they fulfilled at least five criteria.

Studies comparing MAL-PDT and cryotherapy were not able to fulfill three criteria because they were not double blind, and the assessment of the outcome was not blinded as well. There were minimal numbers lost to follow-up reported in the studies ranging from 0 to 17%.

Table 1. Detailed descriptions of eligible studies included in the review

First author (year) Study type	Comparator group	Study size	Patients treated with MAL-PDT, %	Primary aims	Population criteria
Szeimies [17], (2002) Multicenter, open, randomized, controlled study	Cryotherapy (1 session MAL-PDT vs. double freeze-thaw cryotherapy)	202 patients 732 lesions (367 treated with MAL-PDT) Follow-up: 3 months	50.5	Lesion CR, cosmetic outcomes, and patient satisfaction	Age: >18 years M:F T = 66:36 C = 58:42 ≤10 AK lesions
Kaufmann [26], (2008) Multicenter, randomized, intraindividual trial	Cryotherapy (1 session of MAL PDT vs. single freeze-thaw cryotherapy with non-CR lesions retreated at week 12)	121 patients 1,343 lesions Follow-up: 24 weeks	100	Lesion response, cosmetic outcomes, patient preferences, and safety	Age: ≥18 years Patients with non-hyperkeratotic AKs 98% located on the extremities, the rest on the trunk and neck M:F = 78:43 ≥4 comparable symmetrical AKs of similar severity on both sides of the body
Morton [31] (2006) Multicenter, randomized, intraindividual study	Cryotherapy (1 session of MAL-PDT vs. double freeze-thaw cryotherapy with non-CR lesions retreated at week 12)	119 patients 1,501 lesions Follow-up: 24 weeks	100	Lesion response, cosmetic outcomes, and patient satisfaction	Age: ≥18 years M:F = 108:11 Diagnosed with non-hyperkeratotic AKs on face and scalp AK of similar severity and number on both sides of the face and scalp
Freeman [25] (2003) Multicenter, prospective, randomized, controlled study	Cryotherapy and placebo (2 sessions of MAL-PDT or placebo PDT, 7 days apart, vs. single freeze-thaw cryotherapy)	200 patients 855 lesions (295 treated with MAL-PDT) Follow-up: 3 months	43.1	CR and cosmetic outcomes, patient satisfaction, and tolerability	Age: ≥18 years M:F T = 49:39 C = 54:35 P = 16:7 Mild-to-moderate nonpigmented AKs of the face and scalp
Pariser [27] (2003) Multicenter, randomized, double-blind, placebo-controlled study	Placebo (2 sessions of MAL-PDT or placebo PDT, 7 days apart)	80 patients 502 lesions (260 treated with MAL-PDT) Follow-up: 3 months	52.5	CR rate, cosmetic outcomes, and patient satisfaction	Age: ≥18 years with 4–10 previously untreated mild-to-moderate nonpigmented AKs on the face and scalp M:F T = 36:6 P = 34:4

Table 1. Continued

First author (year) Study type	Comparator group	Study size	Patients treated with MAL-PDT, %	Primary aims	Population criteria
Braathen [32] (2008) Multicenter, randomized, parallel-group open study	Short (1-hour) and long (3-hour) incubation period and low (80 mg/g) and high (160 mg/g) concentration cream	112 patients 384 lesions Follow-up: 3 and 12 months	100	CR rate, lesion recurrence rate, and cosmetic outcomes	Age: 43–91 years M:F = 63:49 Most lesions located on the scalp
Pariser [24] (2008) Multicenter, randomized, double-blind study	Placebo (2 sessions of MAL-PDT or placebo PDT, 7 days apart)	96 patients 723 lesions (363 treated with MAL-PDT) Follow-up: 3 months	51	CR rate, lesion recurrence rate, and cosmetic outcomes	Age: ≥18 years M:F T = 42:7 P = 37:10 4–10 nonpigmented, untreated AK lesions on the face and scalp
Szeimies [23] (2009) Multicenter, double-blind randomized, placebo-controlled study	Placebo (2 sessions of MAL-PDT or placebo PDT, 7 days apart)	115 patients 832 lesions (418 treated with MAL-PDT) Follow-up: 3 months	49.6	CR	Age: ≥18 years M:F T = 46:12 P = 45:13 4-10 nonpigmented, untreated AK lesions on the face and scalp
Caekelbergh [22] (2006) Multicenter, randomized, controlled, clinical trial	Cryotherapy	177 patients 781 lesions (360 treated with MAL-PDT) Follow-up: 12 months	49.7	Cost-effectiveness based on efficacy (CR)	Patients with AK lesions
Moloney [28] (2007) Single-center, split-scalp, comparison study	ALA-PDT [one side of scalp treated with ALA (5-hour incubation) or MAL (3-hour incubation) with other side treated with other treatment 2 weeks later]	15 patients 240 lesions	100	Lesion response rate, side effects, and patient preference	Age 59–87 years with extensive scalp AKs
Tarstedt [18] (2005) Multicenter, randomized study	Interval between treatments (1 or 2 treatments with 1 week apart)	211 patients 400 lesions Follow-up: 3 months	100	Lesion response rate, cosmetic effects and adverse effects	Age: ≥18 years with up to 10 clinically diagnosed AK lesions on the face and scalp M:F = 82:129
Rubel [44] (2014) Multicenter, randomized, intraindividual study	Daylight PDT vs. conventional MAL-PDT	100 patients 2,751 lesions	100	Lesion response rate, pain, and subject satisfaction	Age: ≥18 years with mild AKs (grade I) – at least 5 AKs/treatment field (8 × 18 cm) M:F = 75:25

Table 1. Continued

First author (year) Study type	Comparator group	Study size	Patients treated with MAL-PDT, %	Primary aims	Population criteria
Zane [36] (2014) Single-center, randomized, intraindividual, open-label study	Diclofenac 3% in hyaluronic acid gel BD for 90 days vs. conventional MAL-PDT single treatment repeated at 3 months if non-CR	200 patients 1,674 lesions T = 100 patients with 869 AKs D = 100 patients with 805 AKs	50	Lesion response rate, patient CR rate, cosmetic outcome, patient overall satisfaction, and cost-effectiveness	Age: ≥18 years with at least 5 AK lesions on the face and scalp M:F T = 66:34 D = 76:24
Sotiriou [37] (2015) Single-center, intraindividual, open-label, evaluator-blinded study	Imiquimod 5% cream 3 times per week for 4 weeks – 2 courses with 2-week interval between vs. conventional MAL-PDT – 2 sessions 7 days apart	44	100	Number of new lesions, safety, tolerability, and patient preference	Age: ≥18 years with multiple AK lesions on the face and scalp within a 50-cm^2 area M:F = 37:7
Neittaanmäki-Perttu [29] (2014) Single-center, randomized, split-face, observer-blinded study	ALA nanoemulsion (BF-200) vs. daylight MAL-PDT Grade I lesions treated once, grade II–III treated twice	13	100	Lesion response rate, pain, and patient satisfaction	Age: ≥18 years and older
Ko [30] (2014) Single-center study	ALA 6 h and halogen lamp at 150 J/cm^2 vs. conventional MAL-PDT	58 T = 29 patients with 69 AK lesions A = 29 patients with 153 AK lesions	50	Lesion response rate, recurrence rates, cosmetic outcomes, and adverse events	2–10 facial AKs M:F T = 10:19 A = 5:24
Fargnoli [43] (2015) Single-center randomized, intraindividual study	Daylight PDT vs. conventional MAL-PDT	35	100	Lesion response rate, pain, and patient satisfaction	Adults with face or scalp AKs
Wiegell [45] (2012) Multicenter, randomized study	Daylight PDT 1.5 vs. 2.5 h of daylight exposure	145 2,768 AK lesions	100	Lesion response rate	Adults with at least 5 AKs within 25-cm^2 of the face or scalp M:F = 117:28

M:F = Male female ratio; T = treatment/MAL-PDT group; P = placebo group; C = cryotherapy group; D = diclofenac group; A = ALA group.

Table 2. Methodological quality of the included studies

First author (year)	Allocation concealment	Participants' blinding status	Investigators' blinding status	Lesion assessment blinding status	Intention-to-treat analysis	Loss to follow-up, %
Szeimies [17] (2002)	Yes	Not blinded	Not blinded	Not blinded	Yes	4.45
Kaufmann [26] (2008)	Yes	Not blinded	Not blinded	Not blinded	Yes	3.30
Morton [31] (2006)	Yes	Not blinded	Not blinded	Not blinded	Yes	5.04
Freeman [25] (2003)	Yes	Blinded for placebo and not blinded for cryotherapy	Blinded for placebo and not blinded forcryotherapy	Blinded for placebo and not blinded for cryotherapy	Yes	10.78
Pariser [24] (2008)	Yes	Blinded	Blinded	Blinded	Yes	0.00
Pariser [27] (2003)	Yes	Blinded	Blinded	Blinded	Yes	3.75
Braathen [32] (2008)	Yes	Not blinded	Not blinded	Not blinded	Yes	16.97
Caekelbergh [22] (2006)	Yes	Not blinded	Not blinded	Not blinded	Yes	0.00
Szeimies [23] (2009)	Yes	Blinded	Blinded	Blinded	Yes	12.98
Moloney [28] (2007)	Yes	Blinded	Blinded	Blinded	Yes	6.25
Tarstedt [18] (2005)	Yes	Not blinded	Not blinded	Not blinded	Yes	2.84
Rubel [44] (2014)	Yes	Not blinded	Blinded	Blinded	Yes	3
Zane [36] (2014)	Yes	Not blinded	Blinded	Blinded	Yes	2
Sotiriou [37] (2015)	Yes	Not blinded	Blinded	Blinded	No	12
Neittaanmäki-Perttu [29] (2014)	Yes	Not blinded	Blinded	Blinded	Yes	0.00
Ko [30] (2014)	Yes	Not blinded	Blinded	Blinded	Yes	0.00
Fargnoli [43] (2015)	Yes	Not blinded	Blinded	Blinded	Yes	0.00
Wiegell [45] (2012)	Yes	Not blinded	Blinded	Blinded	Yes	2.06

Results of Included Studies

There is now a large body of evidence to support the use of MAL-PDT for AK treatment. Table 3 shows the results of the included studies. The studies might have another primary aim but data extracted were focused on the three outcomes reported in this review.

All the studies showed significant results in evaluating the efficacy of topical MAL-PDT compared to placebo cream. Three-month (lesion) CR rates for MAL-PDT are consistently high at around 90% (for two treatment sessions).

Of all the studies, Szeimies et al. [23] reported lower patient CR rates after a single PDT: 68% with MAL-PDT and 7% with placebo PDT compared with 82 and 21%, respectively, in the study conducted by Pariser et al. [24] and 80 and 18%, respectively, from the prospective randomized study carried out by Freeman et al. [25]. The latter two studies examined response after two treatment sessions 1 week apart. Tarstedt et al. [18] found that a single treatment with MAL-PDT, repeated after 3 months only for nonresponding lesions, was as effective as routinely using two treatments (7 days apart). MAL-PDT is now licensed for AK using a single treatment, repeated after 3 months only when necessary.

The result is slightly different in comparison with cryotherapy where the efficacy of both treatments was almost similar. The efficacy favored cryotherapy if the lesion of AK was on the extremities, as reported by Kaufman et al. [26] (88 vs. 78%). Other studies which involved lesions on the face and scalp were consistently showing the same result which favored MAL-PDT over cryotherapy.

AKs often appear in cosmetically sensitive areas such as the face. Since field cancerization is a highly treatable condition, cosmetic outcome is an important consideration, and PDT may offer a significant advantage over alternative therapies in this respect. As summarized in table 3, a number of phase III studies evaluating MAL-PDT in AK have provided a consistently favorable cosmetic outcome, rating outcome after MAL-PDT as 'excellent' or 'good' by 96, 97 and 98% of investigators, respectively [17, 25, 27].

All the studies showed that MAL-PDT provided a consistently favorable cosmetic outcome, rated as excellent by the investigators. For example, Freeman et al. [25] and Szeimies et al. [17] demonstrated that the cosmetic outcome with MAL-PDT was significantly superior to that achieved with cryotherapy 3 months after treatment (84 vs. 51% reporting 'excellent cosmetic outcome' in the Australian multicenter study and 96 vs. 81% reporting outcome 'excellent' or 'good' in the European multicenter study, respectively).

The first study comparing MAL-PDT with ALA-PDT showed slightly better efficacy for MAL-PDT with CR in 47% in comparison to 40% in ALA-PDT [28]. However, the significance of this study was the pain intensity recorded, which was extremely high with ALA-PDT. The more recent studies tended to favor slightly better lesion response rates, but pain intensity remained higher with conventional ALA-PDT [29, 30].

Comparing treatment regimens, both single and double doses have almost similar efficacy. Similarly, treatment intervals (1 or 3 h between cream application) and illumination have minimal difference in efficacy.

Table 3. Results of the included studies

First author (year)	Results		
	lesion response	cosmetic outcomes	side effects
Szeimies [17] (2002)	3-month lesion CR favored (nonsignificantly) cryotherapy 75.3 vs. 68.7%	Excellent or good cosmetic outcomes favored MAL-PDT: 96 vs. 81% (investigators) and 98 vs. 91% (patients)	43% MAL-PDT vs. 26% cryotherapy Burning sensation, skin pain
Kaufmann [26] (2008)	Inferior efficacy for MAL-PDT compared to cryotherapy (78 vs. 88%)	Excellent cosmetic outcomes favored MAL-PDT (79 vs. 56%) Patients preferred MAL-PDT (59 vs. 25%)	Adverse effects: MAL-PDT (43 vs. 62%)
Morton [31] (2006)	CR favored MAL-PDT [week 24 (after retreatment of non-CR lesions at week 12): 86 vs. 83%; week 12: 87 vs. 76%]	Excellent cosmetic outcomes favored MAL-PDT (77 vs. 50%)	Fewer adverse effects with MAL-PDT in comparison to cryotherapy (62.2 vs. 72.3%)
Caekelbergh [22] (2006)	CR favored MAL-PDT (80.7 vs. 57.3%)	Excellent cosmetic outcome for MAL-PDT over cryotherapy (83 vs. 51%)	n.r.
Freeman [25] (2003)	LRR favored MAL-PDT over placebo and cryotherapy: 91 vs. 68 vs. 30%	Excellent cosmetic outcome: 84 vs. 51% by investigators and 76 vs. 56% by patients	Mild-to-moderate local phototoxicity reaction
Pariser [24] (2008)	LRR favored MAL-PDT (86.2 vs. 52.2%) CR favored MAL-PDT (59.2 vs. 14.9%)	Not investigated	MAL-PDT group: mild-to-moderate severity (erythema, skin burning sensation, and pain)
Pariser [27] (2003)	LRR higher for MAL-PDT (89 vs. 38%) CR higher in MAL-PDT with 82 vs. 21%	Excellent cosmetic outcomes in >90% of patients treated with MAL-PDT	Local phototoxicity reactions such as burning sensation, erythema, crusting, and pain
Braathen [32] (2008)	LRR slightly higher using 3 hour incubation period (85 vs. 76% with 1 h, 160 mg/g, 74% with 1 h, 80 mg/g and 77% with 3 h, 80 mg/g) CR: 78% for thin AKs, 74% for thick AKs after 1 h vs. 96 and 87% for 3 h	>75% had excellent cosmetic outcomes	Most were of mild intensity (erythema, pruritus, and pain and burning sensation of the skin)

Table 3. Continued

First author (year)	Results		
	lesion response	cosmetic outcomes	side effects
Szeimies [23] (2009)	LRR favor MAL-PDT: 83.3 vs. 28.7% CR favor MAL-PDT: 68.4 vs. 6.9%	Not investigated	Adverse events: pain of the skin: 55 vs. 22% Erythema: 52 vs. 5% Skin burning sensation: 36 vs. 12%
Moloney [28] (2007)	CR slightly higher in MAL-PDT than ALA-PDT (46.7 vs. 40%)	Not investigated	Pain scores higher for ALA-PDT 10/15 than MAL-PDT 2/15
Tarstedt [18] (2005)	LRR was almost similar (81% for single treatment vs. 87% for double treatment) CR was almost similar (89% for single vs. 80% for double treatment)	Cosmetic outcomes excellent for 75% of the lesions in each treatment group	Adverse effects reported in 45% patients (burning sensation of the skin, pain, erythema mostly of mild-to-moderate intensity and relatively short duration)
Rubel [44] (2014)	3-month lesion CR 88.9% c-MAL-PDT vs. 85.3% DL-MAL-PDT Mild AKs 89.9 vs. 86.4%	90% good or excellent	Adverse events 59% c-PDT, 39% DL-PDT Pain: 5.7±2.3 vs. 0.8±1.2, respectively
Zane [36] (2014)	3-month lesion CR 85.9% with MAL-PDT and 51.8% with DHA ($p < 0.0001$) AKs of all thicknesses were significantly more responsive to MAL-PDT Patient CR rates at 3 months were 68% with MAL-PDT and 27% with DHA 12-month patient CR 37% with MAL-PDT and 7% with DHA	Investigator assessment Excellent 64% MAL, 17% DHA Good 31% MAL, 75% DHA Patient assessment Excellent 70% MAL, 28% DHA Good 25% MAL, 68% DHA	MAL-PDT: pain all patients – VAS 4.8±1.4 Erythema, edema, blisters, and crusts 100% DHA: mild-to-moderate erythema with itching/burning sensation 84%
Sotiriou [37] (2015)	No difference in numbers of new lesions appearing	n.r.	MAL: pain 100%, erythema 100%, edema 65.9%, erosions and crusting 25% Imiquimod: erythema 100%, scaling 50.2%, erosions and crusting 34.1%, edema 7.1%, and ulceration 7.1%
Neittaanmäki-Perttu [29] (2014)	At 3 months BF-200 ALA cleared 71/84 (84.5%) and MAL 69/93 (74.2%) of the AKs ($p = 0.099$), all grades responding equally	No difference in patient preference	Both treatments were nearly painless with similar adverse reactions

Table 3. Continued

First author (year)	Results		
	lesion response	cosmetic outcomes	side effects
Ko [30] (2014)	At 3 months, lesion CR comparable between the ALA-PDT and MAL-PDT (68.0 vs. 62.3%; p = 0.410) At 6 months, lesion CR was 63.4% for ALA-PDT and 56.5% for MAL-PDT (p = 0.441) At 12 months, lesion CRs were similar in the ALA-PDT and MAL-PDT groups (55.0 vs. 45.1%; p = 0.395)	Excellent or good 89.6% of patients who received ALA-PDT 96.5% of patients who received MAL-PDT	MAL-PDT caused significantly less pain than ALA-PDT (p = 0.005), with a median VAS score of 3.4±2.0 and 5.0±2.4, respectively All patients reported adverse events at the treatment site Most common types of reactions were erythema (ALA, 75.8%; MAL, 72.4%), burning sensation (ALA, 79.3%; MAL, 65.5%), hyperpigmentation (ALA, 72.4%; MAL, 65.5%), crust formation (ALA, 69.0%; MAL, 55.2%), pruritus (ALA, 31.0%; MAL, 24.1%), edema (ALA, 20.7%; MAL, 7.0%), and bullae (ALA, 10.3%; MAL, 7.0%)
Fargnoli [43] (2015)	No difference in CR rate of AK I at 3 months between DL-PDT and c-PDT (87 vs. 91%; RR = 0.96; p = 0.16) Lower CR rate with DL-PDT than with c-PDT for AK II (36 vs. 61%; RR = 0.58, p = 0.06) and III (25 vs. 46%; RR = 0.50, p = 0.20)	n.r.	DL-PDT was better tolerated being associated with lower pain and occurrence of fewer adverse events
Wiegell [45] (2012)	3-month lesion CR no difference between 1.5- and 2.5-hour exposure Mean lesion response grade I 75.9%, grade II 61.2%, grade III 49.1%	n.r.	n.r.

c- = Conventional; DHA = diclofenac in hyaluronic acid gel; DL- = daylight; LRR = lesion response rate; n.r. = not reported.

For the side effect evaluation, all the studies reported similar side effects of MAL-PDT, which was mostly a skin burning sensation, pain in the skin, and skin erythema. In comparison with cryotherapy, the results were inconsistent: Szeimies et al. [17] reported higher side effects for MAL-PDT, while Morton et al. [31] and Kaufman et al. [26] documented fewer side effects for MAL-PDT. However, the side effects reported were well tolerated.

Discussion

Methodological Analysis
Table 2 shows that only the study by Pariser et al. [24] fulfilled all the criteria for a high-quality study. All studies (100%) chosen in this review performed allocation concealment. This method minimizes selection bias because subjects were randomized to be allocated to treatment or control groups. Studies that compared MAL-PDT with cryotherapy were not blinded for both investigator and subjects because of the methodological differences.

Studies which have minimal patients lost to follow-up are able to minimize attrition bias. In this review, studies by Pariser et al. [24] and Caekelbergh et al. [22] documented 0% loss to follow-up. The highest percentage of loss to follow-up (17%) was reported by Braathen et al. [32].

Studies by Kaufman et al. [26] and Morton et al. [31] had an intraindividual study design. This type of study is powerful as it can minimize interindividual variation, which may exist if the procedure is performed in different patients. For example, in this study, the patients had a similar opinion towards the level of side effects they suffered for each of the treatments.

Placebo-Controlled Studies
The results reported in all 3 studies comparing MAL-PDT and placebo cream demonstrated that MAL-PDT is an appropriate treatment for multiple AK lesions based on the lesion CR rate. There is a high observed placebo response in some studies relative to MAL-PDT. Patient CR rates were also high in all these studies, which further strengthens the evidence of its good efficacy. The cosmetic outcomes between placebo and MAL cream have no significant differences as the procedure does not really differ in the two groups, and assessment was only performed on lesions that demonstrated CR. However, reported adverse effects were higher in MAL-PDT than placebo PDT, with frequent erythema, skin burning, and pain.

Cryotherapy-Controlled Studies
There was insufficient evidence to prove that the efficacy of MAL-PDT is better than cryotherapy for all lesions from the studies chosen in this review. This is due to the fact that the location of the lesions resulted in different response rates. For example,

lesions on the extremities showed almost similar efficacy with slight favoring of cryotherapy over MAL-PDT, as discussed by Kaufmann et al. [26]. Other evidence showed that efficacy is better in AK lesions located on the face and scalp. This is supported by the study conducted by Kurwa et al. [33] suggesting that the AK lesions on the extremities might be more resistant than on the face and scalp. Kaufmann et al. [26] also discussed that the resistance might be due to the low amount of pilosebaceous glands on the extremities, which can reduce the absorption of MAL cream. However, regarding cosmetic outcomes in terms of patient and doctor preference, MAL-PDT was superior to cryotherapy in all the studies included. Cryotherapy caused scarring and depigmentation of the skin at the treatment site and the surrounding lesion. In contrast, MAL-PDT conserves the healthy skin. In terms of side effects, both treatments were safe and well tolerated. The incidence of adverse effects of MAL-PDT were consistent in all the studies with skin burning, pain, and erythema listed as frequent symptoms experienced by the patients. However, the adverse effects were reported as mild to moderate, and they were well tolerated by the subjects.

Aminolevulic Acid-Photodynamic Therapy-Controlled Studies
Results showed that both ALA-PDT and MAL-PDT were effective in the treatment of AKs on the face and scalp. Almost similar numbers in AK lesion reduction were achieved with both treatments. However, pain intensity was reported higher on ALA-PDT-treated sites. There is only one study available that directly compared ALA-PDT and MAL-PDT. One theory postulates that ALA causes more pain because it is transported by γ-aminobutyric acid receptors present in peripheral nerve endings [34]. Because MAL-PDT produces slightly better efficacy and less pain intensity, most patients preferred to undergo MAL-PDT treatment rather than ALA-PDT.

A randomized, split-face, prospective, observer-blinded study in 13 patients with 177 AKs compared ALA nanoemulsion (BF-200 ALA) with MAL daylight PDT. Grade I AKs were treated once and grade II–III AKs were treated twice, with the topical photosensitizer layer being 0.25 mm thick. Seventy-one of the 84 AKs cleared with BF-200 ALA and 69 of 93 AKs treated with MAL cleared (84.5 vs. 74.2%, $p = 0.099$). No difference in patient preference was reported, and both treatments were nearly painless with similar adverse reaction profiles [29].

In a study by Ko et al. [30], 58 patients with 222 facial AKs were treated with topical PDT: 153 lesions in 29 patients with ALA and 69 lesions in 29 patients with MAL, with incubations periods of 6 and 3 h, respectively, followed by illumination with a halogen lamp (150 J/cm^2) and an LED lamp (37 J/cm^2), respectively. Similar response rates of 56.9 and 50.7%, respectively, were reported at 12 months. In addition to there being no statistical difference in recurrence/cure rates, there was no difference in cosmetic outcome between both photosensitizers at the 6- and 12-month follow-ups.

Regimen Comparison Study

The recommended regimen of MAL-PDT is a 3-hour incubation with 160 mg/g MAL before illumination. This review was not intended to investigate the dose and treatment interval but to investigate the efficacy of MAL-PDT. Results were consistent between previously reported studies, and reaffirm the efficacy and tolerability of MAL-PDT. However, it is interesting to note that Braathen et al. [32] pointed out 1-hour incubation with 160 mg/g MAL appeared to be nearly as effective as the recommended 3-hour incubation (CR 76% for 1 h vs. 85% for 3 h).

Tarstedt et al. [18] reported that MAL-PDT was effective either with one or two treatment sessions 1 week apart (CR 89% for single vs. 80% for double treatment). They suggested that single treatment is sufficient to treat AKs but advised to conduct two treatments for thick AK lesions.

Ablative fractional laser therapy prior to application of ALA or MAL enhanced porphyrin fluorescence of both photosensitizers particularly at short time points (30 min) compared with 3 h [35].

A comparison of conventional MAL-PDT with diclofenac 3% in hyaluronic acid gel in 200 patients with 1,674 AKs showed clearance rates of 85.8 and 51.8%, respectively, at 3 months. Patient CR rates were 68 and 27% at 3 months, respectively, which reduced to 37 and 7% at 12 months, respectively. Both treatment groups reported very good or excellent cosmetic outcome. Cost-effective analysis reporting costs per patient with CR favored MAL-PDT at 3 and 12 months [36].

Forty-four patients with actinic damage of face or scalp were randomized in a split-face manner to treatment with MAL-PDT or imiquimod 5%. The number of participants developing new lesions in the treated field, the primary endpoint, showed no difference during the 12 month follow up [37].

Limitations and Conclusions

Limitations and Future Research Directions

This review has several limitations. MAL-PDT is well established but often still considered a new treatment, which was only approved by the FDA in 2004. Studies investigating its efficacy and cosmetic outcomes are limited. For example, there are only limited published studies that compare MAL-PDT and ALA-PDT. Similarly, studies involving lesions on the extremities are also limited. Most of the studies involved AK lesions on the face or scalp.

Another weakness of this review was that it did not compare the type of lesions between studies. For example, it did not compare the percentage of CRs in thin and thick lesions. It is important to consider this issue because thin lesions may give better CR rates than thick lesions. Therefore, some studies, which reported higher CR rates, might consist of more subjects with thin lesions. However, this was rarely reported in the studies included in this review.

Finally, this review did not compare MAL-PDT with topical 5-fluorouracil treatment. It is well known that 5-fluorouracil provides better short-term economic outcomes in comparison to MAL-PDT. However, it usually involves wide areas of AK lesions. Studies available for review comparing MAL-PDT and 5-fluorouracil dealt with BCC and Bowen's disease, but not AK treatment.

More research should be conducted in order for us to strengthen the existing evidence. Therefore, dermatologists can recommend MAL-PDT as a first-line treatment and provide strong evidence to the patient.

Conclusion

Of the various treatment comparisons from the studies included in this review, MAL-PDT is particularly well suited for the treatment of AKs as it offers high cure rates and minimal side effects. Moreover, it has excellent cosmetic outcomes in comparison to cryotherapy, as well as generally well-tolerated local adverse effects, and is therefore suitable for the treatment of AK lesions, particularly on the face and scalp. Perhaps most importantly, PDT can be used over large surface areas and therefore may be suitable for the treatment of multiple AK lesions and areas of 'field cancerization' (fig. 1, 2).

Future research directed towards investigating MAL-PDT for lesions on other areas of the body and comparing MAL-PDT with other topical field treatments such as 5-fluorouracil should be conducted.

Daylight Photodynamic Therapy with Methyl Aminolevulinate

A new method of PDT for AKs is the use of natural daylight as the illumination source. A number of consensus statements, including Spanish-Portuguese [38], Australian [39], European [40], and International ones [41], have recommended daylight-mediated MAL-PDT, which involves preparation of the treatment field, application of broad-spectrum, nonphysical blocker sunscreen, application of MAL 0.1–0.2 mm thick, followed by 2 h of daylight exposure, commencing within 30 min of MAL application. It is not recommended to be performed when the temperature is below 10°C or excessively high, nor when it is raining. MAL is applied to the treatment field without occlusion. In sunny environments such as Australia, there is adequate daylight throughout the year to conduct PDT utilizing this technique [42]. The benefits of this technique are the reduction in pain and the absence of a need for specialized equipment. It also dramatically reduces the time required for patients to be in the clinic.

A recent Italian paper [43] (involving 35 patients using an intrapatient left-right comparison) demonstrated no difference in CR rate in AK grade I at 3 months: 87 vs. 91%, (RR = 0.96, p = 0.16) for daylight and conventional PDT, respectively. For AK grade II (moderate thickness), a lower CR rate was noted with daylight PDT than con-

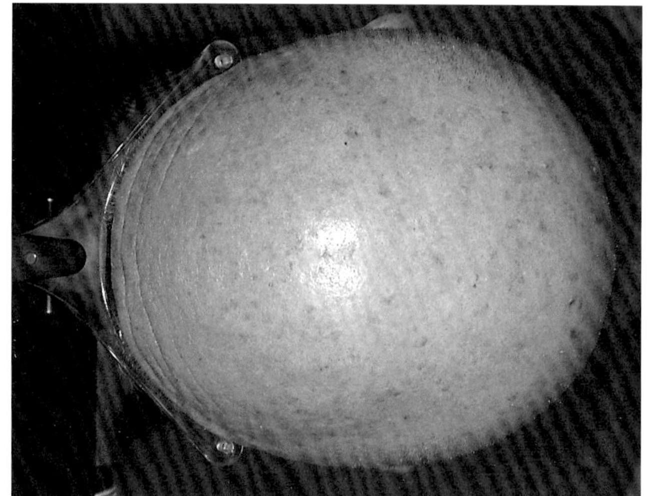

Fig. 1. Typical 'field cancerization' changes (scalp) suitable for MAL-PDT.

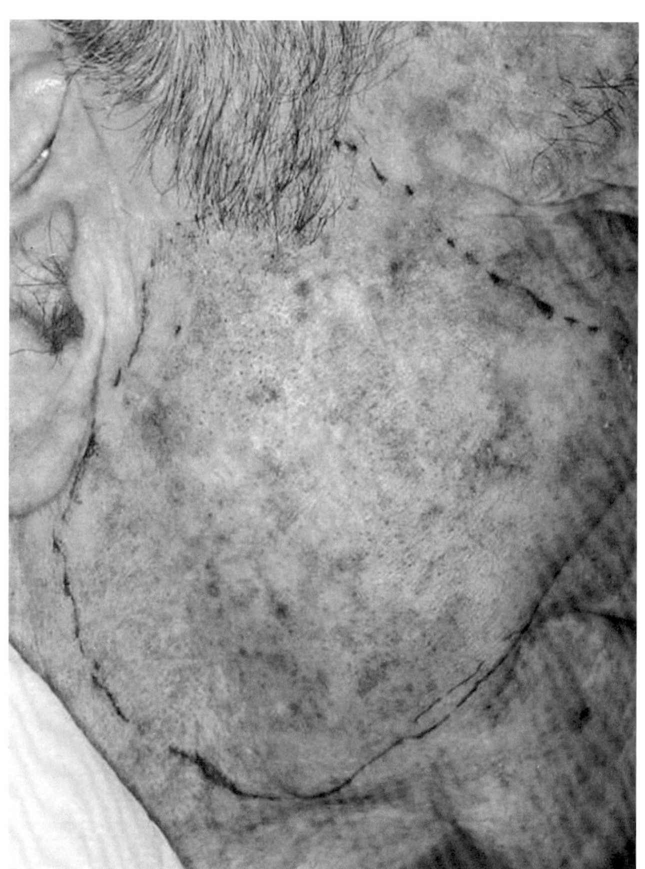

Fig. 2. Typical 'field cancerization' changes (cheek) suitable for MAL-PDT.

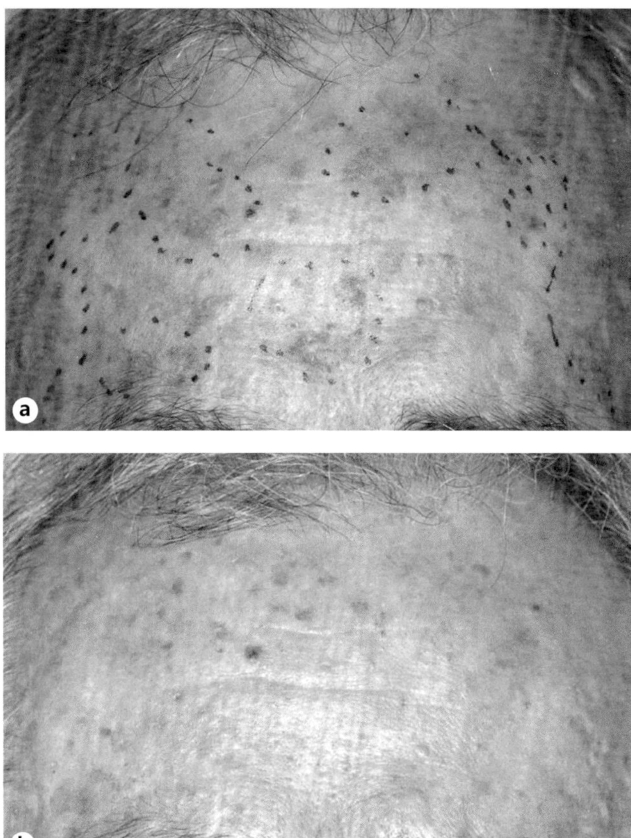

Fig. 3. Multiple AKs (forehead) before (**a**) and 3 months after (**b**) MAL-PDT.

ventional PDT (36 vs. 61%, respectively; RR = 0.58, $p = 0.06$). At the 6-month review, recurrence rate was slightly higher for daylight PDT (17 vs. 12%, respectively; RR = 1.0, $p < 0.5$). Adverse effects of pain and local inflammation severity were lower in the daylight PDT side.

One hundred patients with face or scalp AKs participated in a controlled, randomized, investigator-blinded, multicenter, intraindividual study comparing daylight PDT and conventional PDT. Twelve weeks after a single treatment session, the lesion response rate was 89.2% for daylight PDT, noninferior to 92.8% for conventional PDT. At 24 weeks, 96% of mild lesions remained in remission. The advantage of daylight PDT was a significantly lower pain score (0.8 vs. 5.7 on a 10-point scale, $p < 0.001$) with better tolerability and higher participant satisfaction [44].

In a study by Wiegell et al. [45], 145 participants with 2,769 AKs on the face and scalp were treated with MAL-PDT, using 1.5 or 2.5 h of daylight exposure to activate the protoporphyrin formed. There was no difference in response rates between the two incubation periods. Moderate-to-thick AKs were less effectively treated with lower CR rates, but most were reduced to a lower grade at 3 months with a single treatment (fig. 3–5).

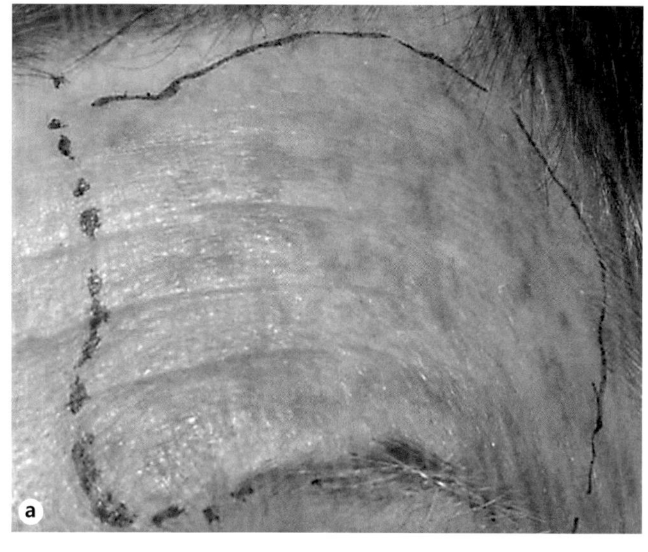

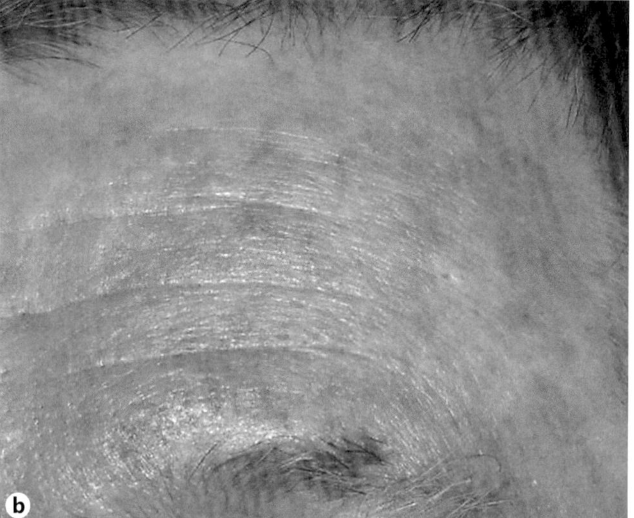

Fig. 4. Multiple AKs (forehead) before (**a**) and 3 months after (**b**) MAL-PDT.

Photodynamic Therapy with Methyl Aminolevulinate for Photorejuvenation

PDT is an evolving treatment for photodamage with considerable benefits and less downtime compared to ablative resurfacing [46]. Topical PDT has been reported to be effective in inducing improvement in global scores for photoaging, lentigines/mottled hyperpigmentation, tactile skin roughness, fine lines/wrinkles, and sallow complexion [46–48]. The clinical benefits are thought to be at least in part due to histologically proven upregulation of collagen production and decreased elastotic material in the dermis, and increased epidermal proliferation. It is thought that cytokine induction secondary to PDT induces neocollagenesis [46, 47].

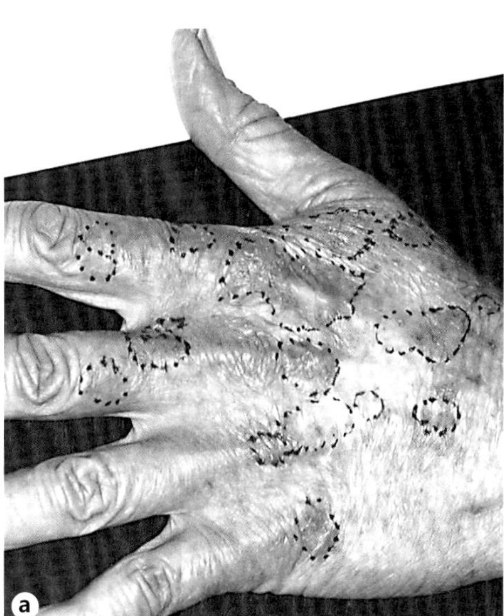

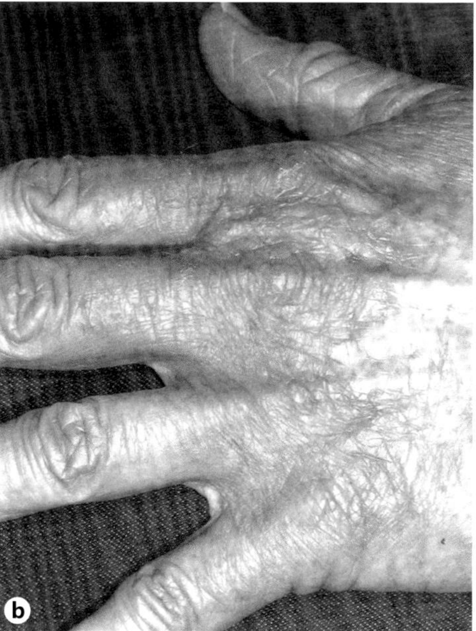

Fig. 5. Multiple AKs (left hand) before (**a**) and 3 months after (**b**) MAL-PDT.

Numerous clinical studies have confirmed the observation that in trials with standard PDT for AK arising within areas of photodamaged skin, the signs of skin aging were markedly improved as positive and desirable side effects [47, 48].

UV radiation in sunlight induces reactive oxygen species within the skin, resulting in increased transcription of matrix metalloproteinases and decreased procollagen 1 and 3 gene expression, which in turn results in diminished dermal matrix generation. Accumulation of degraded collagen in the dermis, as a result of UV radiation, also antagonizes neocollagenesis [46]. UV radiation-induced changes in the skin include elastosis along with collagen degeneration and decrease, and manifest clinically as sallowness and coarse wrinkles. Sun exposure also results in pigmentary dyschromias including freckles, lentigines, and mottled hyperpigmentation. Neoangiogenesis results in telangiectasia formation [46].

The most frequently used assessment tool for signs of skin aging is a 5-point score (0–4) looking at fine lines, mottled pigmentation, sallowness, tactile roughness, telangiectasia, coarse wrinkles, facial erythema, sebaceous gland hyperplasia, and global score. Improvement in fine lines and tactile roughness, increased skin smoothness, improvement in elastosis and skin color, and reduction in hyperpigmentation have been reported. Coarse wrinkles and sebaceous gland hyperplasia seem less likely to improve. Telangiectasia and mottled hyperpigmentation seem to particularly improve with intense pulsed light (IPL) or pulsed dye laser treatment (PDL).

IPL without photosensitizer is capable of improving telangiectasia, fine wrinkles, and age spots [49]. The combination of IPL with MAL has been demonstrated in a number of studies using split-face comparison to be superior. For PDT trials, polychromatic light from IPL (in the range of 500–1,300 nm) is used with a cutoff filter allowing transmission of light above 600 nm, and pulse duration is typically set in the millisecond range. PDT with IPL is perceived to be less painful than with continuous irradiation with red light [50]. Many of the studies examining photodynamic photorejuvenation have utilized 20% ALA and IPL devices. Such studies will not be discussed further in this chapter, other than to say these studies have resulted in improvement in fine lines and mottled pigmentation, but no enhancement with ALA of effectiveness of IPL on sallowness and tactile roughness [51, 52].

PDLs have been used for PDT of nonmelanoma skin cancers with efficacy equivalent to noncoherent light sources, with lower pain experienced [53]. Studies using ALA with PDLs have been used to manage photodamage with resultant increased softness, improved texture but no added improvement in vascular irregularities [46, 54]. ALA has also been used in combination with blue light for photoaging with improvement in skin quality, fine lines, and sallowness reported [55].

In many countries, red light is most commonly used for PDT. This is due to the excellent depth of penetration and licensing approval [47]. Most of the studies (albeit small in number) using incoherent red light PDT for photoaging, have used MAL. A study by Kuijpers et al. [56] showed no difference in short-term efficacy or side effects between ALA and MAL. Kasche et al. [57] demonstrated MAL induced less pain than ALA and was better tolerated.

Zane et al. [58] used MAL with red light (LED at 37 J/cm^2) for severe photodamage, demonstrating significant improvement for mottled pigmentation, fine lines, sallowness, and roughness. No benefit was seen for coarse/deep lines/wrinkles, facial erythema, telangiectasia, and sebaceous gland hyperplasia [48].

Issa et al. [59] reported improvement in wrinkles, skin texture, and skin firmness following two sessions of MAL-PDT, 4 weeks apart. MAL was incubated for 2 h under plastic occlusion. Illumination was with noncoherent red light (LED; 635 nm, 37 J/cm^2). Global clinical improvement was noted in 10 of 14 participants. Improvement was greater at 6 than at 3 months.

It would appear that to obtain satisfactory results with MAL-PDT for photorejuvenation, a 3-hour incubation time is required [46]. Ruiz-Rodriguez et al. [60] performed a split-face study using MAL-PDT with red light and reported moderate improvement in tactile roughness, fine wrinkles, skin tightness, and skin smoothness to be more marked with 3- than 1-hour incubation time. Pigment changes and telangiectasia were unaltered. This was at the cost of local edema, erythema, and scaling, which occurred to a greater extent.

Sanclemente et al. [61], in a split-face study with two treatment sessions of Metvix PDT 2–3 weeks apart using a 3-hour incubation time and the Aktilite, reported improvement in global signs of skin aging, roughness, dyspigmentation, fine lines, sallowness, and erythema, but no improvement in telangiectasia. Patient satisfaction was reported to be 80.4%.

Using the Atktilite and MAL, Szeimies et al. [62] showed significant improvement regarding skin aging, fine lines, sallowness, roughness, erythema, telangiectasia, and hyperpigmentation, but not in wrinkles. Erythema, edema, crusts, and erosions were reported as side effects.

Ten patients with photodamage and multiple AKs treated with MAL-PDT showed an improvement in overall skin appearance, texture, elasticity, and superficial wrinkling. Discrete lesions had MAL applied for 3 h, whilst the intratreatment field had only 1 h of incubation. Illumination was with red light (Aktilite). Eight patients had a single session, the other 2 had a second session 2 days later. Clinical improvement in mottled hyperpigmentation, fine lines, roughness, sallowness, and photoaging were seen in all patients. This assessment was performed 1 month after therapy [63].

In a split-face study, Ruiz-Rodriguez et al. [64] showed enhanced improvement in mild-to-moderate fine lines/superficial wrinkles/rhytides (but without AKs) in the perioral region and subject satisfaction scores after MAL-PDT (3-hour incubation) with Aktilite in combination with nonablative fractional laser thermolysis (2 sessions, 3 weeks apart) than with fractional laser alone, when assessed 4 and 12 weeks after treatment. Unfortunately, erythema and scarring were more common with the combination than with fractional laser alone.

In patients with photodamage and multiple AKs, the addition of microneedles 1.5 mm in length after Metvix application was compared with conventional MAL-PDT (incubation 90 min, illumination red LED lamp). Microneedling alone showed improvement in fine lines at 30 days, while global scores for mottled pigmentation, roughness, and sallowness improved by a negligible amount. By 90 days, microneedling also seemed to improve facial erythema and coarse wrinkles. However, pain, crusting, erythema and edema were more common on the microneedle side [65].

In a poster presentation, Caramel et al. reported improvement in hyperpigmentation, fine lines, roughness, and pale skin when assessed 3 months after MAL-PDT (3-hour incubation, Aktilite, 37 J/cm^2 illumination). Fine lines and blemishes improved in 100%, overall quality was assessed as improved in 83%, and 90% of participants were satisfied with results. Less significant improvement was seen in deep wrinkles, erythema, facial telangiectasia, and sebaceous gland hypertrophy. Decreased elastotic material and increased new collagen and elastin fibers were seen histologically.

A number of studies have been undertaken to explore the possible mechanisms of action of MAL-PDT for skin rejuvenation.

Using high-frequency, high-resolution echographic sonography evaluation, Zane et al. [58] demonstrated an increase in skin thickness with thinning of the subepidermal low echogenic band (elastotic material) after MAL-PDT. Issa et al. [59] demonstrated histological skin remodeling in photodamaged skin with a reduction in elastotic fibers and increased collagen fibers 6 months after Metvix PDT treatment.

The selection of the light source for activation of Metvix for photorejuvenation depends on a variety of factors. Palm et al. [66] showed no difference in the degree of improvement following red or blue light after 1 h of MAL incubation in an intrapatient split-area MAL-PDT study. The authors report that both sources improved the appearance of photodamaged skin. However, the majority of patients were also treated with PDL or IPL. Interestingly, the greatest improvements in photodamage measures were in pigmentation. Side effects were mild and not different between the two light sources. Of note, patients were only followed for 30 days.

When lentigines and telangiectasia are present, it would appear appropriate to use IPL or PDL as the activating light source. If AKs are also present, current recommendations would be to use regulatory authority-approved treatment protocols [47, 53].

References

1 Werner RN, Stockfleth E, Connolly SM, Correia O, Erdmann R, Foley P, Gupta AK, Jacobs A, Kerl H, Lim HW, Martin G, Paquet M, Pariser DM, Rosumeck S, Röwert-Huber HJ, Sahota A, Sangueza OP, Shumack S, Sporbeck B, Swanson NA, Torezan L, Nast A: Evidence- and consensus-based (S3) Guidelines for the Treatment of Actinic Keratosis – International League of Dermatological Societies in cooperation with the European Dermatology Forum – short version. J Eur Acad Dermatol Venereol 2015, Epub ahead of print.

2 Salasche SJ: Epidemiology of actinic keratoses and squamous cell carcinoma. J Am Acad Dermatol 2000;42:4–7.

3 Drake LA, Ceilley RI, Cornelison RL: Guidelines of care for actinic keratoses. J Am Acad Dermatol 1995; 32:95–98.

4 Squamous cell carcinoma, actinic keratosis, and seborrheic keratosis; in Sauer GC. Manual of Skin Diseases, ed 5. Philadelphia, Lippincott, 1985.

5 Marks R, Rennie G, Selwood T: The relationship of basal cell carcinomas and squamous cell carcinomas to solar keratoses. Arch Dermatol 1998;124:1039–1042.

6 Glogau RG: The risk of progression to invasive disease. J Am Acad Dermatol 2004;42:23–24.

7 Nelson MA, Einspahr JG, Alberts DS: Analysis of the p53 gene in human precancerous actinic keratosis lesions and squamous cell cancers. Cancer Lett 1994; 85:23–29.

8 Leffell DJ: The scientific basis of skin cancer. J Am Acad Dermatol 2000;42:18–22.

9 de Berker D, McGregor JM, Hughes BR; British Association of Dermatologists Therapy Guidelines and Audit Subcommittee: Guidelines for the management of actinic keratoses. Br J Dermatol 2007;156: 222–230.

10 Parrish JA: Immunosuppression, skin cancer, and ultraviolet A radiation. N Engl J Med 2005;353: 2712–2713.

11 Calzavara-Pinton PG, Venturini M, Sala R: Photodynamic therapy: update 2006. Part 2. Clinical results. J Eur Acad Dermatol Venereol 2007;21:439–451.

12 Angell-Petersen E, Sorensen R, Warloe T, Soler AM, Moan J, Peng Q, et al: Porphyrin formation in actinic keratosis and basal cell carcinoma after topical application of methyl 5-aminolevulinate. J Invest Dermatol 2005;126:265–271.

13 Peng Q, Soler A, Warloe T, Nesland J, Giercksky K: Selective distribution of porphyrins in skin thick basal cell carcinoma after topical application of methyl 5-aminolevulinate. J Photochem Photobiol B 2001;62:140–145.

14 Braathen LR, Szeimies R-M, Basset-Seguin N, Bissonnette R, Foley P, Pariser D, et al: Guidelines on the use of photodynamic therapy for nonmelanoma skin cancer: an international consensus. J Am Acad Dermatol 2007;56:125–143.

15 Gad F, Viau G, Boushira M, Bertrand R, Bissonnette R: Photodynamic therapy with 5-aminolevulinic acid induces apoptosis and caspase activation in malignant T cells. J Cutan Med Surg 2001;5:8–13.

16 Noodt BB, Berg K, Stokke T, Peng Q, Nesland JM: Apoptosis and necrosis induced with light and 5-aminolaevulinic acid-derived protoporphyrin IX. Br J Cancer 1996;74:22–29.

17 Szeimies RM, Karrer S, Radakovic-Fijan S, Tanew A, Calzavara-Pinton PG, Zane C, et al: Photodynamic therapy using topical methyl 5-aminolevulinate compared with cryotherapy for actinic keratosis: a prospective, randomized study. J Am Acad Dermatol 2002;47:258–262.

18 Tarstedt M, Rosdahl I, Berne B, Svanberg K, Wennberg A-M: A randomized multicenter study to compare two treatment regimens of topical methyl aminolevulinate (Metvix)-PDT in actinic keratosis of the face and scalp. Acta Derm Venereol 2005;85:424–428.

19 Wolf JE Jr, Taylor JR, Tschen E, Kang S: Topical 3.0% diclofenac in 2.5% hyaluronan gel in the treatment of actinic keratoses. Int J Dermatol 2001;40:709–713.

20 Gold MH: Pharmacoeconomic analysis of the treatment of multiple actinic keratoses. J Drugs Dermatol 2008;7:23–25.

21 Morton CA, Wulf HC, Szeimies RM, Gilaberte Y, Basset-Seguin N, Sotiriou E, Piaserico S, Hunger RE, Baharlou S, Sidoroff A, Braathen LR: Practical approach to the use of daylight photodynamic therapy with topical methyl aminolevulinate for actinic keratosis: a European consensus. J Eur Acad Dermatol Venereol 2015;29:1718–1723.

22 Caekelbergh K, Annemans L, Lambert J, Roelandts R: Economic evaluation of methyl aminolaevulinate-based photodynamic therapy in the management of actinic keratosis and basal cell carcinoma. Br J Dermatol 2006;155:784–790.

23 Szeimies RM, Matheson RT, Davis SA, Bhatia AC, Frambach Y, et al: Topical methyl aminolevulinate photodynamic therapy using red light-emitting diode light for multiple actinic keratoses: a randomized study. Dermatol Surg 2009;35:586–592.

24 Pariser D, Loss R, Jarratt M, Abramovits W, Spencer J, Geronemus R, et al: Topical methyl-aminolevulinate photodynamic therapy using red light-emitting diode light for treatment of multiple actinic keratoses: a randomized, double-blind placebo-controlled study. J Am Acad Dermatol 2008;59:569–576.

25 Freeman M, Vinciullo C, Francis D, Spelman L, Nguyen R, Fergin P, et al: A comparison of photodynamic therapy using topical methyl aminolevulinate (Metvix) with single cycle cryotherapy in patients with actinic keratosis: a prospective, randomized study. J Dermatolog Treat 2003;14:99–106.

26 Kaufmann R, Spelman L, Weightman W, Reifenberger J, Szeimies RM, Verhaeghe E, et al: Multicentre intraindividual randomized trial of topical methyl aminolaevulinate photodynamic therapy vs. cryotherapy for multiple actinic keratoses on the extremities. Br J Dermatol 2008;158:994–999.

27 Pariser DM, Lowe NJ, Stewart DM, Jarratt MT, Lucky AW, Pariser RJ, et al: Photodynamic therapy with topical methyl aminolevulinate for actinic keratosis: results of a prospective randomized multicenter trial. J Am Acad Dermatol 2003;48:227–232.

28 Moloney FJ, Collins P: Randomized, double-blind, prospective study to compare topical 5-aminolaevulinic acid methylester with topical 5-aminolaevulinic acid photodynamic therapy for extensive scalp actinic keratosis. Br J Dermatol 2007;157:87–91.

29 Neittaanmäki-Perttu N, Karppinen TT, Grönroos M, Tani TT, Snellman E: Daylight photodynamic therapy for actinic keratoses: a randomized double-blinded nonsponsored prospective study comparing 5-aminolaevulinic acid nanoemulsion (BF-200) with methyl-5-aminolaevulinate. Br J Dermatol 2014;171:1172–1180.

30 Ko DY, Kim KH, Song KH: Comparative study of photodynamic therapy with topical methyl aminolevulinate versus 5-aminolevulinic acid for facial actinic keratosis with long-term follow-up. Ann Dermatol 2014;26:321–331.

31 Morton C, Campbell S, Gupta G, Keohane S, Lear J, Zaki I, et al: Intraindividual, right-left comparison of topical methyl aminolaevulinate-photodynamic therapy and cryotherapy in subjects with actinic keratoses: a multicentre, randomized controlled study. Br J Dermatol 2006;5:1029–1036.

32 Braathen LR, Paredes BE, Saksela O, Fritsch C, Gardlo K, Morken T, et al: Short incubation with methyl aminolevulinate for photodynamic therapy of actinic keratoses. J Eur Acad Dermatol Venereol 2008;23:550–555.

33 Kurwa HA, Yong-Gee SA, Seed PT, Markey AC, Barlow RJ: A randomized paired comparison of photodynamic therapy and topical 5-fluorouracil in the treatment of actinic keratosis. J Am Acad Dermatol 1999;41:414–418.

34 Rud E, Gederaas O, Hogset A, Berg K: 5-Aminolevulinic acid, but not 5-aminolevulinic esters, is transported into adenocarcinoma cells by system BETA transporters. Photochem Photobiol 2000;71:640–647.

35 Haedersdal M, Sakamoto FH, Farinelli WA, Doukas AG, Tam J, Anderson RR: Pretreatment with ablative fractional laser changes kinetics and biodistribution of topical 5-aminolevulinic acid (ALA) and methyl aminolevulinate (MAL). Lasers Surg Med 2014;46:462–469.

36 Zane C, Facchinetti E, Rossi MT, Specchia C, Calzavara-Pinton PG: A randomized clinical trial of photodynamic therapy with methyl aminolaevulinate vs. diclofenac 3% plus hyaluronic acid gel for the treatment of multiple actinic keratoses of the face and scalp. Br J Dermatol 2014;170:1143–1150.

37 Sotiriou E, Apalla Z, Vrani F, Lallas A, Chovarda E, Ioannides D: Photodynamic therapy vs. imiquimod 5% cream as skin cancer preventive strategies in patients with field changes: a randomized intraindividual comparison study. J Eur Acad Dermatol Venereol 2015;29:325–329.

38 Gilaberte Y, Aguilar M, Almagro M, Correia O, Guillén C, Harto A, Pérez-García B, Pérez-Pérez L, Redondo P, Sánchez-Carpintero I, Serra-Guillén C, Valladares LM: Spanish-Portuguese consensus statement on use of daylight-mediated photodynamic therapy with methyl aminolevulinate in the treatment of actinic keratosis. Actas Dermosifiliogr 2015; 106:623–631.

39 See JA, Shumack S, Murrell DF, Rubel DM, Fernández-Peñas P, Salmon R, Hewitt D, Foley P, Spelman L: Consensus recommendations on the use of daylight photodynamic therapy with methyl aminolevulinate cream for actinic keratoses in Australia. Australas J Dermatol 2015, DOI: 10.1111/ajd.12354.

40 Morton CA, Wulf HC, Szeimies RM, Gilaberte Y, Basset-Seguin N, Sotiriou E, Piaserico S, Hunger RE, Baharlou S, Sidoroff A, Braathen LR: Practical approach to the use of daylight photodynamic therapy with topical methyl aminolevulinate for actinic keratosis: a European consensus. J Eur Acad Dermatol Venereol 2015;29:1718–1723.

41 Wiegell SR, Wulf HC, Szeimies RM, Basset-Seguin N, Bissonnette R, Gerritsen MJ, Gilaberte Y, Calzavara-Pinton P, Morton CA, Sidoroff A, Braathen LR: Daylight photodynamic therapy for actinic keratosis: an international consensus: International Society for Photodynamic Therapy in Dermatology. J Eur Acad Dermatol Venereol 2012;26:673–679.

42 Spelman L, Rubel D, Murrell DF, See JA, Hewitt D, Foley P, Salmon R, Kerob D, Pascual T, Shumack S, Fernandez-Penas P: Treatment of face and scalp solar (actinic) keratosis with daylight-mediated photodynamic therapy is possible throughout the year in Australia: evidence from a clinical and meteorological study. Australas J Dermatol 2015, DOI: 10.1111/ajd.12295.

43 Fargnoli MC, Piccioni A, Neri L, Tambone S, Pellegrini C, Peris K: Conventional vs. daylight methyl aminolevulinate photodynamic therapy for actinic keratosis of the face and scalp: an intra-patient, prospective, comparison study in Italy. J Eur Acad Dermatol Venereol 2015;29:1926–1932.

44 Rubel DM, Spelman L, Murrell DF, See JA, Hewitt D, Foley P, Bosc C, Kerob D, Kerrouche N, Wulf HC, Shumack S: Daylight photodynamic therapy with methyl aminolevulinate cream as a convenient, similarly effective, nearly painless alternative to conventional photodynamic therapy in actinic keratosis treatment: a randomized controlled trial. Br J Dermatol 2014;171:1164–1171.

45 Wiegell SR, Fabricius S, Gniadecka M, Stender IM, Berne B, Kroon S, Andersen BL, Mørk C, Sandberg C, Ibler KS, Jemec GB, Brocks KM, Philipsen PA, Heydenreich J, Hædersdal M, Wulf HC: Daylight-mediated photodynamic therapy of moderate to thick actinic keratoses of the face and scalp: a randomized multicentre study. Br J Dermatol 2012;166: 1327–1332.

46 Kohl E, Torezan LA, Landthaler M, Szeimies RM: Aesthetic effects of topical photodynamic therapy. J Eur Acad Dermatol Venereol 2010;24:1261–1269.

47 Karrer S, Kohl E, Feise K, Hiepe-Wegener D, Lischner S, Philipp-Dormston W, Podda M, Prager W, Walker T, Szeimies RM: Photodynamic therapy for skin rejuvenation: review and summary of the literature – results of a consensus conference of an expert group for aesthetic photodynamic therapy. J Dtsch Dermatol Ges 2013;11:137–148.

48 Calzavara-Pinton P, Arisi M, Sereni E, Ortel B: A critical reappraisal of off-label indications for topical photodynamic therapy with aminolevulinic acid and methylaminolevulinate. Rev Recent Clin Trials 2010; 5:112–116.

49 Babilas P, Schreml S, Landthaler M, Szeimies RM: Inkohärentes Licht in der Dermatologie. Hautarzt 2010;61:153–166.

50 Babilas P, Knobler R, Hummel S, Gottschaller C, Maisch T, Koller M, Landthaler M, Szeimies RM: Variable pulsed light is less painful than light-emitting diodes for topical photodynamic therapy of actinic keratosis: a prospective randomized controlled trial. Br J Dermatol 2007;157:111–117.

51 Dover JS, Bhatia AC, Stewart B, Arndt KA: Topical 5-aminolevulinic acid combined with intense pulsed light in the treatment of photoaging. Arch Dermatol 2005;141:1247–1252.

52 Gold MH, Bradshaw VL, Boring MM, Bridges TM, Biron JA: Split-face comparison of photodynamic therapy with 5-aminolevulinic acid and intense pulsed light versus intense pulsed light alone for photodamage. Dermatol Surg 2006;32:795–801.

53 Karrer S, Bäumler W, Abels C, Hohenleutner U, Landthaler M, Szeimies RM: Long-pulse dye laser for photodynamic therapy: investigations in vitro and in vivo. Lasers Surg Med 1999;25:51–59.

54 Key DJ: Aminolevulinic acid-pulsed dye laser photodynamic therapy for the treatment of photoaging. Cosmet Dermatol 2005;18:31–36.

55 Touma D, Yaar M, Whitehead S, Konnikov N, Gilchrest BA: A trial of short incubation, broad-area photodynamic therapy for facial actinic keratoses and diffuse photodamage. Arch Dermatol 2004;140:33–40.

56 Kuijpers DI, Thissen MR, Thissen CA, Neumann MH: Similar effectiveness of methyl aminolevulinate and 5-aminolevulinate in topical photodynamic therapy for nodular basal cell carcinoma. J Drugs Dermatol 2006;5:642–645.

57 Kasche A, Luderschmidt S, Ring J, Hein R: Photodynamic therapy induces less pain in patients treated with methyl aminolevulinate compared to aminolevulinic acid. J Drugs Dermatol 2006;5:353–356.

58 Zane C, Capezzera R, Sala R, Venturini M, Calzavara-Pinton P: Clinical and echographic analysis of photodynamic therapy using methylaminolevulinate as sensitizer in the treatment of photodamaged facial skin. Lasers Surg Med 2007;39:203–209.

59 Issa MC, Pineiro-Maceira J, Vieira MT, Olej B, Mandarim-de-Lacerda CA, Luiz RR, Manela-Azulay M: Photorejuvenation with topical methyl aminolevulinate and red light: a randomized, prospective, clinical, histopathologic, and morphometric study. Dermatol Surg 2010;36:39–48.

60 Ruiz-Rodriguez R, Lopez L, Candelas D, Pedraz J: Photorejuvenation using topical 5-methyl aminolevulinate and red light. J Drugs Dermatol 2008;7:633–637.

61 Sanclemente G, Medina L, Villa JF, Barrera LM, Garcia HI: A prospective split-face double-blind randomized placebo-controlled trial to assess the efficacy of methyl aminolevulinate + red-light in patients with facial photodamage. J Eur Acad Dermatol Venereol 2011;25:49–58.

62 Szeimies RM, Torezan L, Niwa A, Valente N, Unger P, Kohl E, Schreml S, Babilas P, Karrer S, Festa-Neto C: Clinical, histopathological and immunohistochemical assessment of human skin field cancerization before and after photodynamic therapy. Br J Dermatol 2012;167:150–159.

63 Macedo OR, Bussade M, Fujimura M, et al: Methylaminolevulinate (MAL)-photodynamic therapy (PDT) for the treatment of actinic keratosis (AKs) and photorejuvenation. http://www.derme.com.br/publicacoes/artigos/cong10/.

64 Ruiz-Rodriguez R, López L, Candelas D, Zelickson B: Enhanced efficacy of photodynamic therapy after fractional resurfacing: fractional photodynamic rejuvenation. J Drugs Dermatol 2007;6:818–820.

65 Torezan L, Chaves Y, Niwa A, Sanches JA Jr, Festa-Neto C, Szeimies RM: A pilot split-face study comparing conventional methyl aminolevulinate-photodynamic therapy (PDT) with microneedling-assisted PDT on actinically damaged skin. Dermatol Surg 2013;39:1197–1201.

66 Palm MD, Goldman MP: Safety and efficacy comparison of blue versus red light sources for photodynamic therapy using methyl aminolevulinate in photodamaged skin. J Drugs Dermatol 2011;10:53–60.

Peter Foley, MD, FACD
St. Vincent's Hospital Melbourne
41 Victoria Parade
Fitzroy, VIC 3065 (Australia)
E-Mail Peter.FOLEY@svha.org.au

Gold MH (ed): Cosmetic Photodynamic Therapy. Aesthet Dermatol. Basel, Karger, 2016, vol 3, pp 64–84
DOI: 10.1159/000441511

Photodynamic Therapy – Novel Cosmetic Approaches

Girish S. Munavalli[a, b] · Matteo Tretti Clementoni[c] · Marc B. Roscher[d]

[a]Dermatology, Laser, and Vein Specialists of the Carolinas, Charlotte, N.C., and [b]Department of Dermatology, Wake Forest University School of Medicine, Winston-Salem, N.C., USA; [c]Istituto Dermatologico Europeo, Plastic Surgery, Milan, Italy; [d]Department of Dermatology, Nelson R Mandela School of Medicine, Durban, South Africa

Abstract

Photodynamic therapy (PDT) has been evolving from a traditionally medical intervention to a powerful, safe, and efficacious therapy for a wide variety of cosmetic scenarios. Here in this chapter, adjunctive methods are described to enhance the effect of PDT through the use of boosting transepidermal penetration. This has implications for both enhanced therapeutic and enhanced cosmetic effects. It is the authors who wish that readers will find the results compelling and incorporate these simple methods into their own practices.

Introduction

The cosmetic therapy realm is in a constant state of flux, with new technologies and treatment protocols expanding the therapeutic horizons of skin care physicians all over the globe.

Photodynamic therapy (PDT) has been evolving from a traditionally medical intervention to a powerful, safe, and efficacious therapy for a wide variety of cosmetic scenarios.

After the initial 'rediscovery' of PDT in the 60s and beyond, and after the registration of the first commercially available 5-aminolevulinic acid (ALA) product, Levulan, physicians started treating large numbers of patients with short-contact protocols in the office setting. In addition to the expected excellent clearance rates of actinic keratosis (AK), it became patently clear that several additional components of photodamage were also improved [1–4].

Both red and blue light devices are commonly employed light sources in the cosmetic use of PDT, although, more recently, they have been combined with laser devices [5, 6].

Sequential, multidevice usage has evolved towards incorporating the many different and powerful lasers and lights, with each playing a different role in the activation of the photosensitizing agent – and the photodynamic process per se.

Photorejuvenation

Photoaging (also known as dermatoheliosis) generally refers to the accumulated, chronic exposure to ultraviolet (UV) A and UVB light in the spectrum of 290–400 nm, resulting in a prematurely aged cosmetic appearance of the skin [7, 8].

Facial and neck skin are anatomic areas of predilection due to direct, sustained sun exposure. The characteristic clinical signs of this photoaging include fine and coarse wrinkles, roughness, erythema, lentigines, sallowness, and hyperpigmentation. Histologically, epidermal thinning, variable atypia, elastosis, and large irregularly grouped melanocytes are seen.

The targets for photoaged and damaged skin are therefore epidermal, upper and mid-dermal in nature and within the diffusion/action spectrum of ALA and methyl aminolevulinate (MAL).

In addition to inducing mutagenic changes in basal keratinocytes leading to the formation of precancerous AK and cancerous skin lesions, long-term exposure to UV light disrupts the balance between normal collagen production and degradation. UV-irradiated skin favors a pathway of net degradation of dermal type I and III collagen by reduction of procollagen, and possibly an impaired transforming growth factor-β/ Smad pathway [9].

Clinically, this manifests as photoaged skin and differs from sun-protected, naturally aged skin in that it appears thicker, rougher, with coarse/fine wrinkles, and lentiginous mottled pigmentation. The use of ALA-PDT for the successful treatment of nonhyperkeratotic AK is well documented [10].

The concurrent improvement in the photoaged appearance after ALA-PDT has been observed and reported [11–15].

Treatment options for photoaging include chemical peels, topical retinoids, fully ablative and nonablative fractional lasers, intense pulsed light (IPL) and light-emitting diodes (LEDs) [16].

For the purposes of this chapter and PDT-related treatment of photoaging, focus will be on the concurrent use of IPL with PDT, as well as the use of enhanced skin penetration techniques – microneedling, and fractional nonablative and ablative lasers to enhance the effect of PDT. IPL is discussed below.

IPL is a good choice because of its dual functionality as an adjunct photoactivating source, in addition to its inherent properties as a broadband light source for targeting multiple superficial skin chromophores (melanin and hemoglobin).

The use of IPL was a further refinement and expansion on the reach of this procedure to more comprehensively address the full spectrum of photodamaged sequelae.

Ruiz-Rodriguez and López-Rodriguez [17] showed in a series of 17 patients that the use of IPL was safe and effective in treating most of the photodamage components that were found in patients.

Multiple other clinical studies have consistently demonstrated good-to-excellent cosmetic results with the use of PDT. In a prospective, randomized controlled, split-face study, Babilas et al. [18] treated 25 patients with sun-damaged skin treated with MAL followed by irradiation with either an LED (635 nm, 37 J/cm^2) or an IPL device (610–950 nm, 80 J/cm^2). At 3 months, the authors found significant improvement in wrinkling and pigmentation, irrespective of the light source used. Gold et al. [19] evaluated short-contact (30–60 min) ALA-PDT using IPL as a light source, versus IPL alone in 16 patients in a side-by-side design. Patients were exposed to PDT for a total of 3 monthly treatments and followed at months 1 and 3. The IPL treatment parameters were 34 J/cm^2; cutoff filters used were 550 nm for Fitzpatrick skin types I–III and 570 nm for Fitzpatrick skin type IV. They found greater improvement in the ALA-PDT-IPL group compared to IPL alone for all facets of photodamage.

The practical challenge with using PDT for photorejuvenation is the availability of multiple other proven and accepted modalities such as chemical peels, laser, and IPL. The additional time and supply costs of PDT limit it from becoming a widely utilized treatment option for photorejuvenation.

With numerous broadband and single wavelength visible light sources reported to be of benefit in activation of ALA, the following guide below is useful for a starting point [20].

Activate ALA with the appropriate light source(s):

1 Illumination is begun with the pulsed dye laser to individual lesions (if it unavailable, proceed to IPL).
   a 595 nm with a 7-mm spot size, 40-ms pulse width, and 10–12 J/cm^2 (Cynergy; Cynosure, Westford, Mass., USA) with forced cold air cooling (Zimmer; LaserMed, LLC, Shelton, Conn., USA).
   b 595 nm with a 7-mm spot size, 40-ms pulse width, dynamic cooling 30/30, and 10–12 J/cm^2 or Vbeam Perfecta (Syneron Candela, Irvine, Calif., USA).

2 IPL is utilized in non-hair-bearing areas.
   a For skin types I–III, we use the 560-nm cutoff filter and the 590-nm filter for skin types IV (Lumenis 1 or the Lumenis M22; Lumenis Ltd., Yokneam, Israel).
   - If predominant hyperpigmentation (solar lentigines or postinflammatory hyperpigmentation): double pulse technique, 3.0-ms pulse duration for both pulses.
   - If combination of hyperpigmentation (solar lentigines or postinflammatory hyperpigmentation) and erythema: double pulse technique, 3.5-ms pulse duration for both pulses.
   - Predominance of fine telangiectasias: double pulse technique, 4-ms pulse duration for both pulses.

b 10- to 30-ms delay is set between pulses in skin types I–III and 30–40 ms in skin type IV.

c Fluence range of 17–22 J/cm^2, with decreased doses recommended for nonfacial locations.

d Other IPL devices can also be used successfully, though treatment settings must be adjusted appropriately to each device.

3 Finally, simultaneous illumination with blue and red light.

a Blue light source (BluU; DUSA Pharmaceuticals, Inc., Wilmington, Mass., USA) positioned 25–50 mm from the skin, 16 min 40 s, light dose 10 J/cm^2.

b Red light source (Aktilite CL 128; Galderma, Fort Worth, Tex., USA) positioned 50–80 mm from the skin, 8 min 49 s, 37 J/cm^2.

It is important to note that the degree of activation of ALA with different light sources is not equal and not without controversy. It is widely accepted and reported that continuous-wave sources are more effective than pulsed light sources. Blue light is the single best activating wavelength for ALA for AK treatment [21]. Red light is a useful adjunct, but not necessary. Ambient natural sunlight is also used as an adjunct for ALA activation [22].

Enhancing the Photodynamic Therapy Effect

Absorption of ALA and cellular uptake with subsequent conversion to protoporphyrin IX (PpIX) is a prerequisite prior to irradiation with a light source, in order for reactive oxygen species-mediated tissue destruction to take place. The stratum corneum of the epidermis is felt to be the major barrier to passive diffusion of the water-soluble ALA (after topical application) into the basal epidermis and dermis. Shallow penetration of ALA does occur with time; however, short incubation times, focal areas of epidermal hyperkeratosis, the presence of skin surface sebum, and topical cosmetic products can lead to nonuniform absorption and ultimately compromise results. To overcome these obstacles, various strategies have been employed to enhance topical times, curettage, use of chemical penetration enhancers, iontophoresis, microneedling, and microdermabrasion [23, 24].

These strategies are sometimes impractical to employ in a practice with high patient volume because they can be too time consuming (long incubation times, iontophoresis, and microdermabrasion) or because they may be potentially too destructive (curettage) to the skin. Indeed, longer incubation times can result in more pain during treatment, presumably due to increased penetration and uptake at nerve endings [24].

Of these strategies, microneedle devices have the distinct advantage of being simple to use, rapid, well tolerated, bloodless, and relatively low in cost. The use of microneedle rollers for enhancing cosmesis of the face through collagen induction and enhanced penetration of topical cosmeceuticals has been well described [25–27] Interestingly, the use of microneedling rollers, with a needle length of 500 μm has been demonstrated to create numerous transdermal channels and enhance the topical penetration of an optical clearing agent, 95% glycerol, compared to a control. This study alluded to more effective treatment of laser-/light-based devices following this method of optical agent delivery.

As was shown by Henry et al. [28] in 1998, microneedles with only a few hundred microns in length are able effectively penetrate the stratum corneum, which has a thickness of only 10–20 mm. Compared to classical hypodermic needles, these microneedles have the advantage of being relatively painless, although they are inserted at least into the epidermis and sometimes deeper into the superficial dermis where nerves are present. Most likely, their small size reduces the odds of encountering a nerve, or of stimulating it, to produce a painful sensation. Fernandes [25] and Fernandes and Signorini [26] showed that the simple process of wound healing following the targeted use of needling rollers can help to induce dermal collagen remodeling. In a study by Donnelly et al. [23], solid bore, silicon microneedle arrays were able to enhance the delivery of preformed photosensitizers in vivo and in vitro in animal models. Those investigators determined that quantitatively larger amounts of ALA were present in the dermis at depths up to 2 mm (delivered from an occluded ALA patch model) in porcine skin which had underwent needling in comparison to normal porcine skin [28].

The use of needling as a tool for effecting cosmetic improvement in the skin has been widely reported. In early work surrounding the use of microneedling as a way of creating microchannels for the photosensitizer to penetrate deeper into the skin – Kenner and Fernandes – and later Roscher and Fernandes – investigated this technique [Des Fernandes and Marc Roscher, pers. commun].

However, superficial needling with a 0.22-cm device to create microchannels in the impermeable stratum corneum has been investigated for a variety of agents as a penetration-enhancing modality. In this work, it was apparent that the PDT effect was significantly expanded, resulting in persisting erythema and induration (for up to 72 h) – as opposed to the control sides that were treated with PDT alone. A sample protocol for the utilization of microneedling to enhance PDT is detailed at the end of the chapter.

In more recent years, investigators have been assessing ways of improving ALA penetration/absorption into the skin – with a view to improve clinical outcomes and shortening incubation protocols. Enhanced drug delivery has been the focus of interest in recent years, as it has shown that assisted or intensified PDT enhances immunofluorescence patterns as well as the so-called PDT effect. Topical drug delivery is essential to dermatological therapy. However, the cutaneous bioavailability of most topically applied drugs is relatively low with only 1–5% being absorbed into the skin [29].

Unfortunately, some drugs that traverse the epidermis and are absorbed do not penetrate deeply enough to reach the desired target in the tissue [30].

For a topical agent to be active, it must first traverse the rate-limiting outermost barrier of the skin: the stratum corneum. Many medications are too large to penetrate this barrier and require either injectable or systemic delivery. Laser-assisted drug delivery is an evolving modality which may allow for a greater depth of penetration by existing topical medications, more efficient transcutaneous delivery of large drug molecules, and even systemic drug administration via a transcutaneous route.

The use of fractional laser devices to intensify/enhance the PDT effect and resultant clinical outcome was originally proposed by Ruiz-Rodriguez et al. [31] in a series showing safety and efficacy in combination with IPL use and MAL as the photosensitizer.

Building on this concept, investigators undertook evaluation of the impact of fractional CO_2 microchannel enhancement of photosensitizer uptake in an animal model. Fractional CO_2 and Er:YAG lasers (AFXLs) affect the skin barrier by creating vertical, ablated channels using laser wavelengths in the far-infrared spectrum, which are strongly absorbed by tissue water. Experimental in vitro and in vivo porcine studies demonstrated that pretreatment with fractional Er:YAG laser and fractional CO_2 laser facilitates the penetration of topically applied MAL into superficial and deep skin layers, and also promotes an intensified PDT response in superficial and deep dermal compartments [32, 33]. Enhanced fluorescence was achieved and the PDT effect was ostensibly enhanced.

Further studies showed the use of this technique with routine PDT protocols to illustrate superior clinical outcomes than PDT alone. The term intensified PDT has been used for this technique.

It follows then that the combination of this device with PDT has the potential to multiply the cosmetic capacity of both treatments on the proviso that enhanced ALA delivery would be the result, effecting an expanded immunofluorescence reaction and stronger PDT effect [32, 33]. Although there has been some work comparing intensifying approaches, further studies are needed to properly quantify the understanding we have of the concomitant use of this approach in the treatment of photodamage. Better equivocation is required looking at the different intensifying protocols, comparing larger series with investigator-blinded result assessment.

The fact remains that PDT yields remarkable improvement in the different components of photodamage.

When treating with ALA, especially when using techniques that can enhance penetration, effect and response; and light sources that intensify activation (such as IPL and blue light), great detail should be paid to patient care. The use of microneedling rollers and other nonlaser methods as pretreatment and subsequent application of the medication is frequently delegated to nonphysician staff; so it is paramount to follow meticulously planned protocols. What follows are guidelines for achieving the best results, while maximizing patient safety and treatment efficacy.

Techniques and Preoperative Care

After medical or cosmetic indications for PDT have been ascertained, focus should be turned to periprocedural details. It is imperative to obtain a proper patient medical history. Any history of photosensitizing disorders, porphyrias, or documented allergy to ALA or MAL may preclude treatment [34]. Because only visible light is used for activation, concurrent use of medications known to cause toxicity with exposure to UV light is allowed and should not be an issue. Prior history of herpes simplex virus should be elicited and some authors initiate prophylactic measures be taken prior to the initiation of therapy [35]. Skin conditions which promote parakeratotic scale, such as seborrheic dermatitis, should be treated and controlled prior to PDT, as this type of scale is more hyperproliferative and can absorb ALA.

Many methods exist for pretreatment preparation of skin-cleansing regimens. Cleaning allows for a more uniform penetration of ALA and subsequent photoactivation. Acetone is frequently used to degrease the skin and facilitate penetration; however, it has a low flash point, can be painful for open or eroded skin, and its availability may be limited at larger academic institutions. Thus, other cleansing agents are sometimes used. Peikert et al. [36] showed equal degreasing capability between acetone and Hibiclens for prepping skin prior to chemical peeling. Isopropryl alcohol, soaps, α-hydroxy/salicylic acid cleansers, or towelettes can also be used.

After cleansing, numerous techniques (ranging from noninvasive to minimally invasive) can be used to disrupt the stratum corneum and enhance the skin penetration of ALA. The trade-off of several of these methods is added time and expense of supplies as well as staffing. One simple method is gauze abrasion, or the heavy-handed use of 4 × 4 gauze rubbed on the skin. Oscillating brushes or particle/particle-free microdermabrasion have also been reported as methods of enhancement of penetration [36]. The use of microneedling rollers has been studied and shown to promote ALA penetration, absorption, and activation [37]. More recently, fractional nonablative and ablative lasers have been used prior to application to enhance penetration, activation, and efficacy [38].

The application of the topical ALA solution (after mixing per package insert) should be carefully considered. Ideally, the use of the Kerastick (DUSA Pharmaceuticals) cotton-tipped applicator facilitates placement. Application to the full face is best accomplished expressing the solution onto the treatment area and with a gloved hand evenly wiping it over the face in two coats. Care should be taken to apply within close proximity, but be wary of the periorbital areas (including inside the orbital rim). Since actinic damage is frequently present in the lateral/medial brows and into the frontal and sideburn hairlines, these areas should not be overlooked. For nonfacial areas, such as the extremities, occlusion has been used to increase penetration. This can be accomplished with plastic wrap or some other nonporous, flexible material placed over the targeted area after ALA has been applied. Applying a warming blanket can also enhance penetration and increase AK clearance, as demonstrated in a prospective clinical trial [39].

Incubation times will vary and depend on the type of treatment (cosmetic vs. medical), the anatomical area treated, the severity of the actinic damage, and patient tolerance. For the treatment of actinic damage on the face, incubation times of 1–2 h are commonly used in clinical practice. This reduction in treatment time was done primarily for patient and physician convenience as the initial studies had incubation times of 14–18 h which maximized PpIX levels in actinic tissue. On the scalp, typically a minimum of 2 h is used for incubation. A recent multicenter, randomized study found the median AK clearance rate at 12 weeks to be 88.7% for extremities, when treated with ALA under occlusion for 3 h and irradiated with blue light (10 J/cm^2) [40]. These shorter incubation times have resulted in reduced, but acceptable, clearance rates of AKs compared to initial FDA trial data. Incubation should take place in a dark room, devoid of as much ambient light as possible. Typically, discomfort during light treatment will increase with longer incubation times as additional drug is converted to the active form. For this reason as well as cost and patient convenience, many European centers have been conducting 'daylight' PDT, where patients incubate for a much shorter period before spending a few hours outdoors for exposure rather than a device in the clinician's office [40]. Sunscreen is used during this time to prevent UV-induced sunburn since it does not interfere with the visible light activation of PpIX (unless it is applied thickly in an opaque manner). Appropriate exposure times have been developed for various latitudes and weather conditions.

After incubation, the targeted area should be gently washed with water and a cleanser. Irradiation should be carried out in an appropriately sized room preferably without windows and with low ambient light levels (to prevent phototoxicity or photobleaching). The room should also have adequate cooling and ventilation for the light source.

Appropriate eye protection is paramount during all aspects of the procedure to ensure ocular safety. Prolonged exposure to blue and UV light is damaging to the retina [40]. Red light does not seem to result in the same retinal toxicity but ocular protection is still recommended. In the pivotal phase III FDA trial for AK, the fluorescent lamp light source was the BluU (DUSA Pharmaceuticals) with a peak emittance at 417 ± 5 nm and blue-blocking goggles were worn by patients during irradiation [40]. Since a wider variety of light source are used nowadays, the type of goggles used must be suitable to the light source. The preference is for patients to use completely opaque eye protection to minimize exposure. All staff or providers should wear appropriate eyewear prior to entering the room.

Pain during PDT is expected, requiring interventions for pain control including application of ice, use of a fan, interruption of treatment, forced air cooling, and topical and oral analgesia [41]. In the aforementioned study by Touma et al. [11], 3% lidocaine hydrochloride cream topically applied 45 min prior to light exposure offered minimal and statistically insignificant pain control. Because lidocaine is known to provide at least modest pain relief after topical application, the authors felt that the lack of significant benefit probably related to the small sample size, imprecision of the measurement, and inability of patients to compare the active versus vehicle control creams on their skin, since each patient used only one of the preparations.

Cooling adjuncts such as fans and forced air cooling devices are routinely used throughout the treatment to mitigate intraoperative pain and discomfort.

The risk of infection after PDT is exceedingly low. To our knowledge, there are no reports of any reported series of infections occurring after PDT specifically. In our 15-year experience with PDT, treating thousands of patients, we have had less than a 1% infection rate. Exuberant reactions, which result from intense reactions, with denuded skin and oozing should be treated with good topical wound care, including frequent cleansing with soap and water. White vinegar-water soaks (mixed 1:3), performed 2–3 times per day for these reactions, can be a useful adjunct to hydrate the wound and provide a deterrent to infection. If necessary, cephalexin or ciprofloxacin can be used to treat suspected infections empirically, while a culture is pending.

Postoperative Care

Immediately after PDT, patients typically develop erythema to varying degrees, which is sometimes profound in appearance. Edema is also present [37]. Pain tends to subside quickly as the illuminating light source is terminated. Pain is controlled with oral acetaminophen or nonsteroidal anti-inflammatory drugs. For patients with large treatment areas and prolonged incubation times, oral opioid analgesics are sometimes necessary for several days following the procedure. It is very important that patients understand the need for photo avoidance for 24–36 h following treatment.

Covering with opaque clothing is the best way to avoid additional photoreactivity. Use of mineral-based or physical sunblocks (containing zinc oxide or titanium dioxide) is most appropriate for blocking visible light [37]. Most UV-blocking sunscreens that are traditionally used for outdoors will not be sufficient and should not be recommended [37]. If patients feel any tingling or stinging, it is likely that they are being exposed to an ambient light source unknowingly, such as an indoor light or sunlight from a window.

Lastly, different topical protocols have been studied as an adjunct to reduce post-procedural discomfort and erythema. Garcia et al. [42] performed split-face comparisons of four different nonsteroid, over-the-counter products following activation of ALA with pulsed light/blue light. Results were encouraging and showed that the different products all provided some degree of benefit, even though they had different mechanisms of action.

Lastly, the authors have included below a rough protocol for using the microneedling roller with ALA and IPL combined with red light to get effective therapeutic and cosmetic results. This is excerpted from the authors' publication in 2010 that showed statistically significant improvements in photoaging and a reduction in AKs following treatment in a controlled study [43].

Our Methods to Improve the Use of Photodynamic Therapy

The Devices

Roller

The tool is a disposable plastic roller on which very thin and short (300–500 μm in length) needles are mounted. This roller has a handle that permits to move the roller back and forth on the skin.

Intense Pulsed Light

The IPL devices used are the Lumenis 1 or M22 (Lumenis). The devices are equipped with several filters that can be interchanged without changing the head. Additionally, this head is equipped with two cooled sapphire light guides of 15 × 35 and 8 × 15 mm, respectively, that can be used in different anatomical sites. The energy is emitted in a square shape resulting in a more uniform energy emission within each pulse.

Red Light

The red light (630-nm wavelength) device used is the S-630 (Alpha Strumenti, Milan, Italy). The device is composed of a control unit connected to two separate LED emitters. These two emitters have separate power supply and are mounted on two adjustable arms. The emission power is 160 mW/cm^2.

Topical Drug

20% hydrochloride salt of ALA solution (Levulan Kerastick; DUSA Pharmaceuticals) was used.

Indications

All patients presenting a facial photodamage with at least 5 AKs can be submitted to the procedure. The ideal candidate for the procedure is a patient with diffuse facial mottled pigmentations, small telangiectasia, fine lines, tactile roughness of the skin, and several nonhyperkeratotic AKs (fig. 5). Pregnant or nursing women and patients with a history of photosensitivity-related disorders, or presence of an active infectious disease should be excluded.

Treatment Protocol

All patients had to apply a 3% glycolic acid and 3% salicylic acid solution on the face, once a day and during evening, for almost 10 days before the treatment session. They also had to use sun protection for almost 15 days before the same treatment. Eventually still evident hyperkeratotic lesions had to be treated before the procedure by scraping away abnormal tissue using a sharp curette (avoiding bleeding during the maneuver) or could be removed using a more gentle procedure. Therefore, a cotton swab soaked in acetone was placed on top of each lesion and locked in place by a waterproof bandage; 15 min later, this medication could be removed as well as the hyperkeratotic tissue. After accurate cleansing and degreasing (with acetone) of the skin, the roller was passed back and forth on the skin of the face several times. On each aesthetic unit, the roller was used stretching the skin with one hand and handling the roller with the other. The roller was passed back and forth for 5–6 times in one direction before changing it. At the end of this maneuver, the skin had to present a uniform redness without any bleeding. The region of the eyelids was always avoided. The roller was passed on both healthy skin and AK lesions. More aggressive pass-

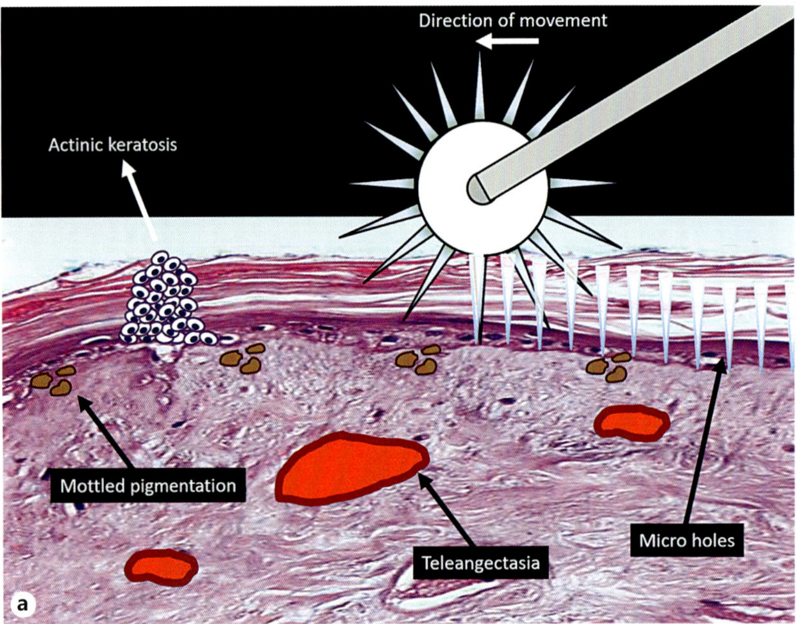

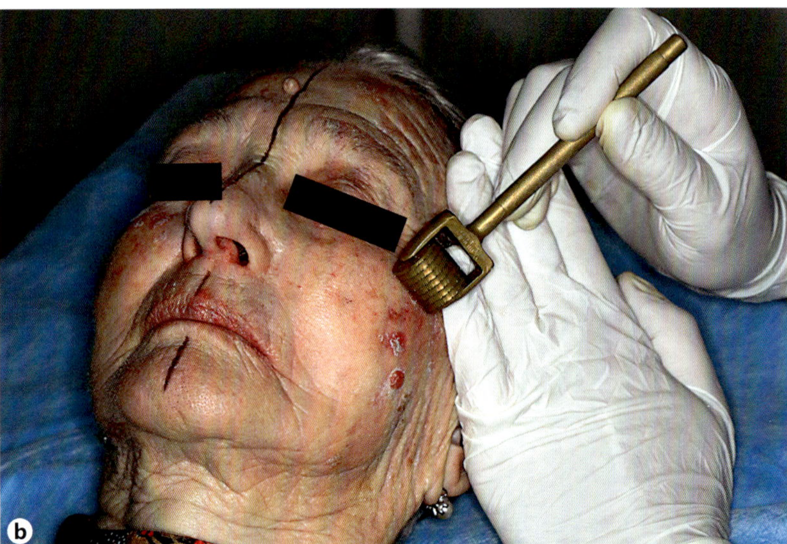

Fig. 1. The roller is passed back and forth on the skin to create thousands of holes. **a** Schematic view. **b** Clinical view.

es (back and forth for 5–6 times in almost 4 different directions) were performed on clinically evident actinic lesions (fig. 1). This part of the treatment is done to create thousands of fine holes that reach and slightly penetrate (due to the needles length) the dermal-epidermal barrier. Through them, each kind of fluid drug can penetrate faster and deeper. Immediately after this mechanic and painless step, ALA was ap-

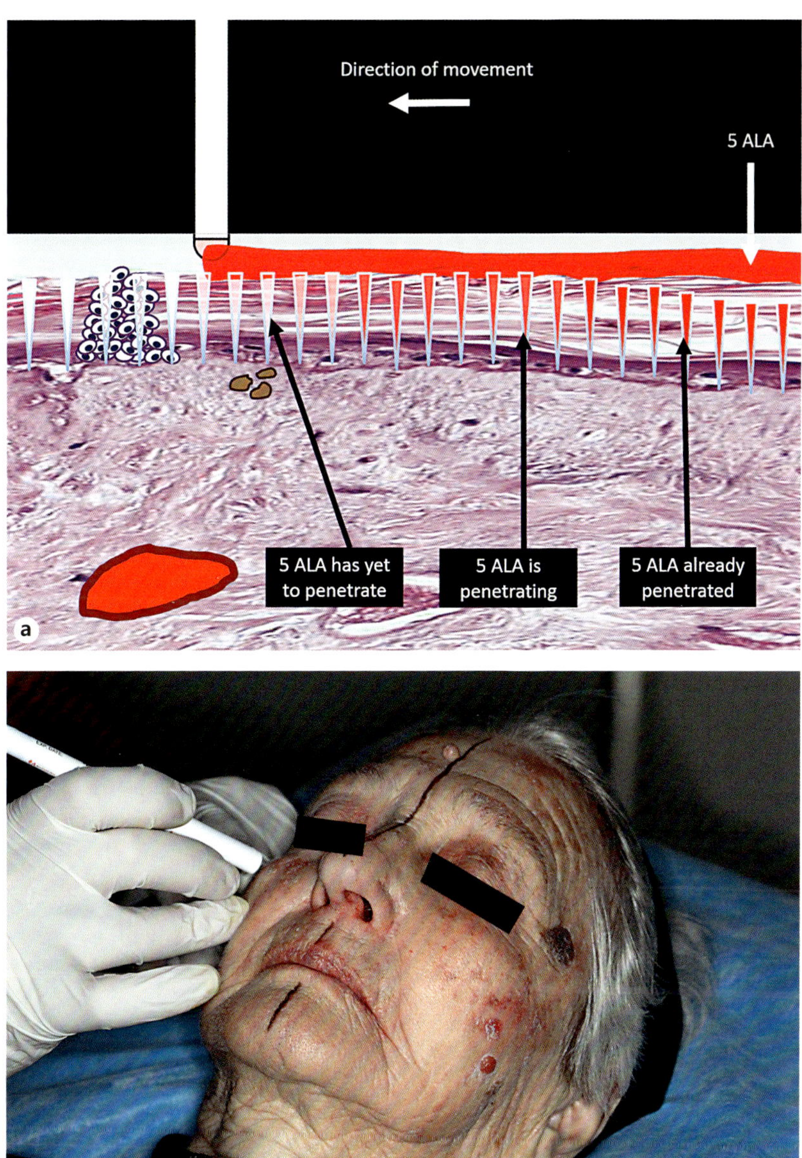

Fig. 2. ALA is applied on the skin, and during the incubation time the drug penetrates the holes allowing the compound to reach the cells faster and deeper thereafter transforming itself into PpIX. **a** Schematic view. **b** Clinical view.

plied on the skin (fig. 2). The ALA solution was initially applied only on clinically evident lesions and then, when the drug has dried (10–15 min), it was applied all over the face. The photosensitizer was left in place for 1 h (actually 60 min on supposedly healthy skin and 75 min on actinic lesions), and then the skin is cleaned using gauzes wet with saline solution. The patient was then submitted to the IPL treatment

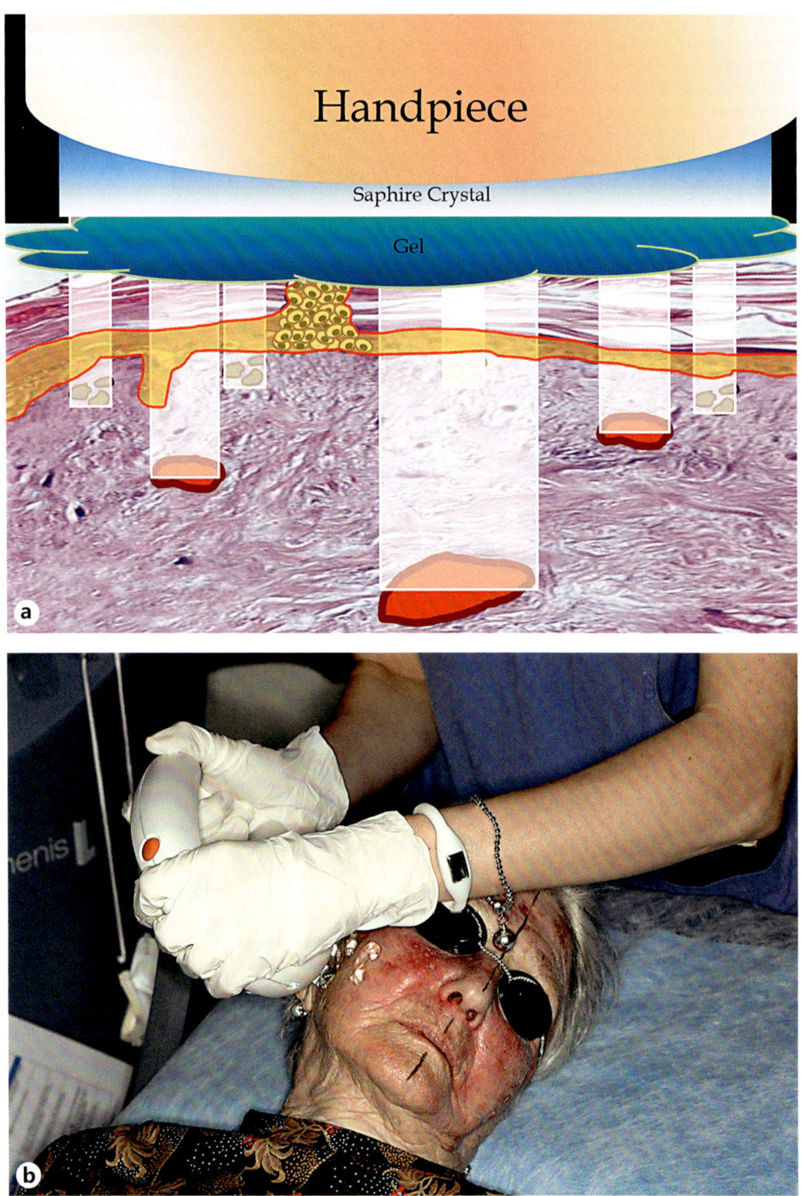

Fig. 3. The IPL treatment reaches the pigmented and vascular targets and partially activates the photodynamic reaction. **a** Schematic view. **b** Clinical view.

(fig. 3). The parameters used were: 560-nm cutoff, 3.0–5.0 ms of double pulse duration, 25–30 ms of delay time, and 19–22 J/cm^2 of fluence. On pigmented lesions, a second pass with a 515-nm cutoff, 3.0/4.0 ms of pulse duration and 14 J/cm^2 of fluence was then performed. The sapphire tip of the IPL handpiece was directly laid on the skin interposing a thin layer of cold water gel covering small anatomical areas.

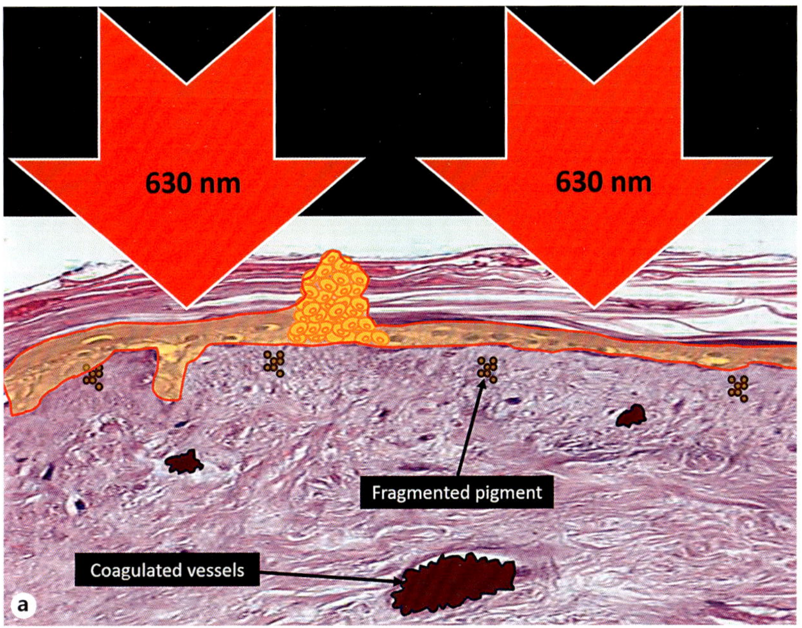

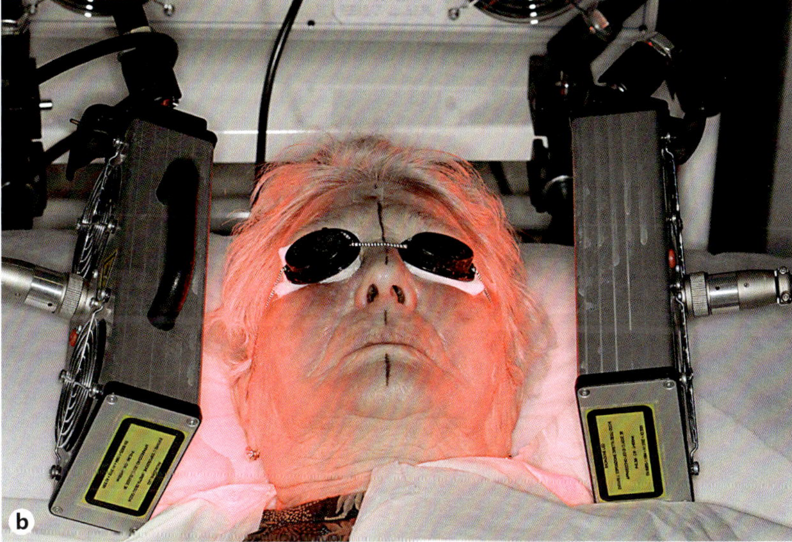

Fig. 4. The LED 630-nm illumination determines a complete photodynamic reaction. **a** Note the coagulated vessels and fragmented pigment. Schematic view. **b** Clinical view.

After the IPL treatment and having accurately removed the gel, the red LED lamp was then used (fig. 4). Moving the adjustable arms of the red light device, the two emitters were placed at a distance of 5 cm from the skin forming a dihedral angle. The light was then switched on for a time (12 min) sufficient to completely activate the photosensitizer. A cold spring water spray helped patients to tolerate the proce-

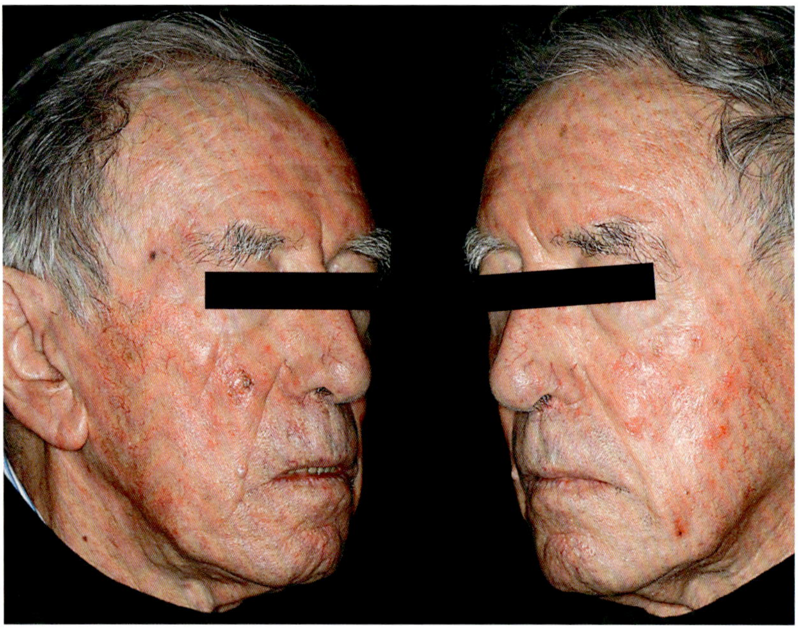

Fig. 5. 69-year-old man before the procedure.

dure. If the patient referred a disturbing itching feeling during the light exposure the light was switched off for 120 s and then switched on again reaching the end of the treatment. The 'on-off-on' treatment permitted to conclude all treatments without any unpleasant sensations by the patients. Protoporphyrin IX emits a red-orange fluorescence when illuminated by a Wood lamp (fig. 6) and the photobleaching effect of the PDT reaction can be used to evaluate the progression of the procedure. At the end of the procedure no orange fluorescence should be observed (fig. 7) on the skin of the patient. Patients were instructed to prevent sun exposure for 48 h after the procedure and advised to apply sunblock with a sun protection factor of 50 or greater three times a day for the following 30 days. After the treatment, patients have to apply a moisturizer at least 4 times a day and they have to keep this regimen for 2 weeks. IPL part of the procedures has melanin granules and fine teleangectasia as targets and only minimally activates the PDT reaction. The PDT reaction is mostly related to the red light illumination (fig. 8).

When the patient presents a lot of aging signs (lentigos and teleangectasia) the IPL part of the procedure is extremely helpfull (fig. 9) to reduce them allowing the operator to achieve a very good outcome (fig. 10).

The combination of the effects of IPL on teleangectasia and lentigos and the new collagen production stimulated by the PDT reaction is able not only to reduce the number and size of AKs (fig. 11) but can give also a nice cosmetic outcome.

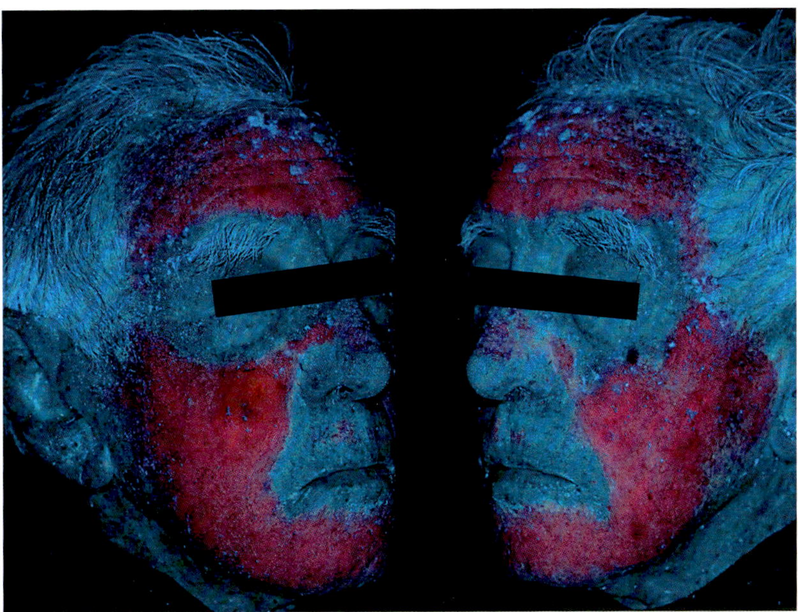

Fig. 6. Fluorescence of the skin of the patient in figure 5 after a 75-min drug incubation.

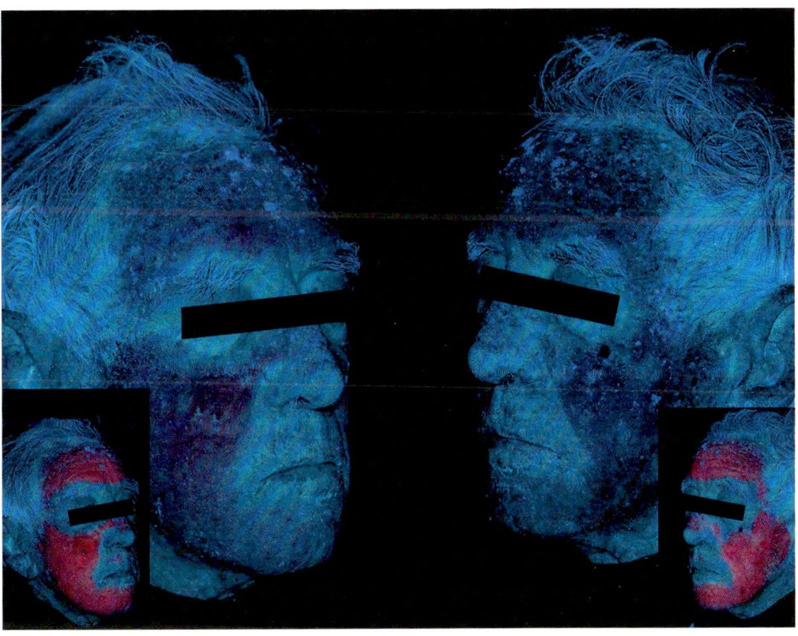

Fig. 7. Patient of figure 5 after the activation of PpIX with IPL and red light. No more fluorescence is evident.

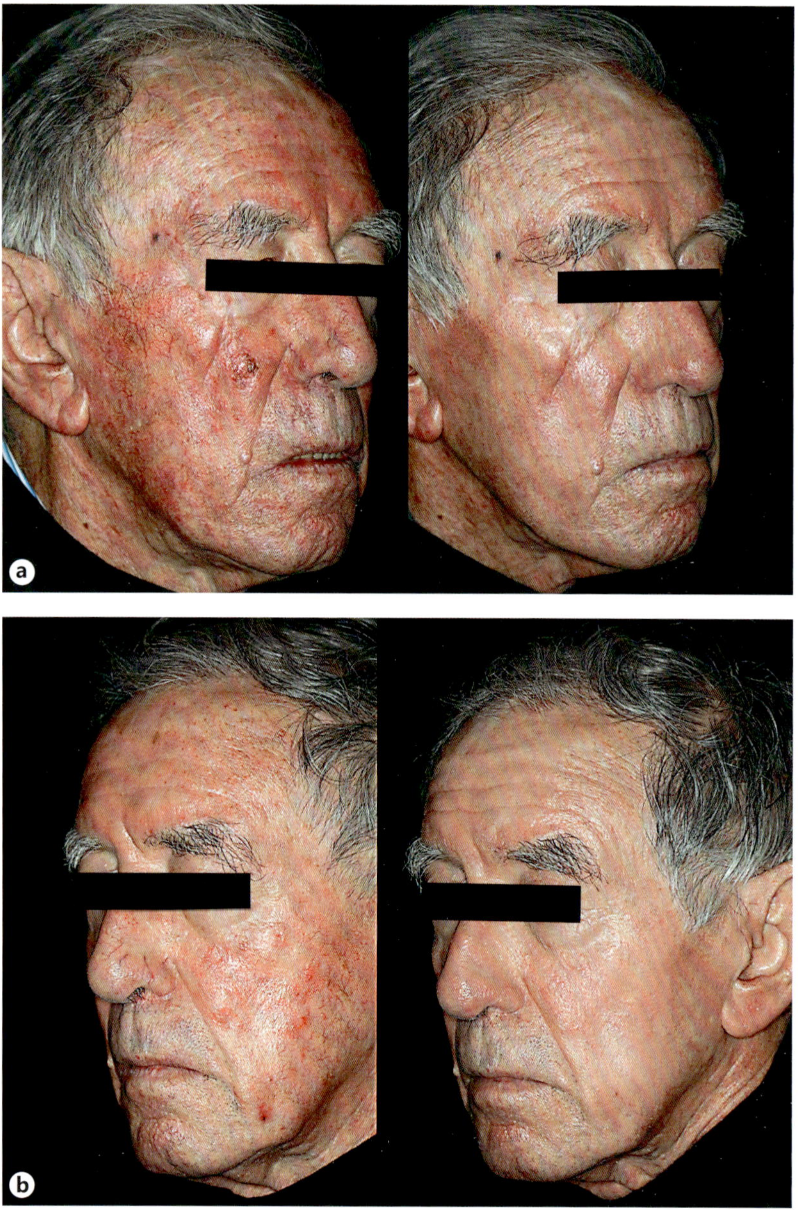

Fig. 8. Patient of figure 5 shown 12 months after the procedure. **a** The right side. **b** The left side.

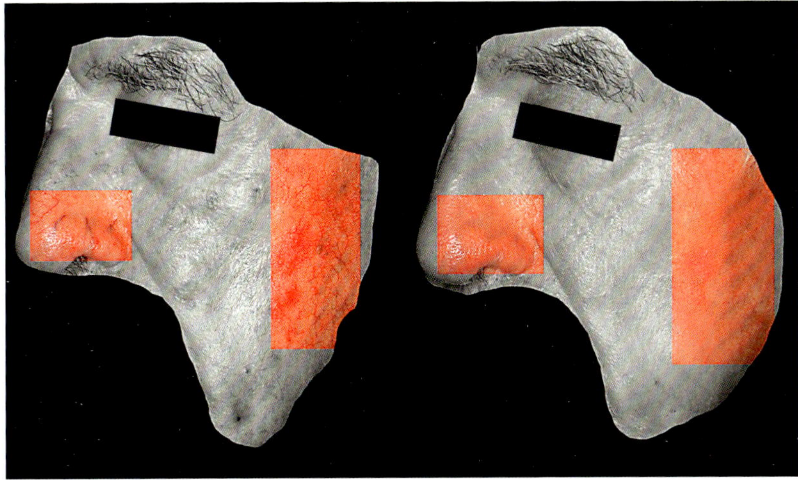

Fig. 9. Fine teleangectasia in 71 year old man before and after the procedure. Blood vessels were completely coagulated and are no more evident.

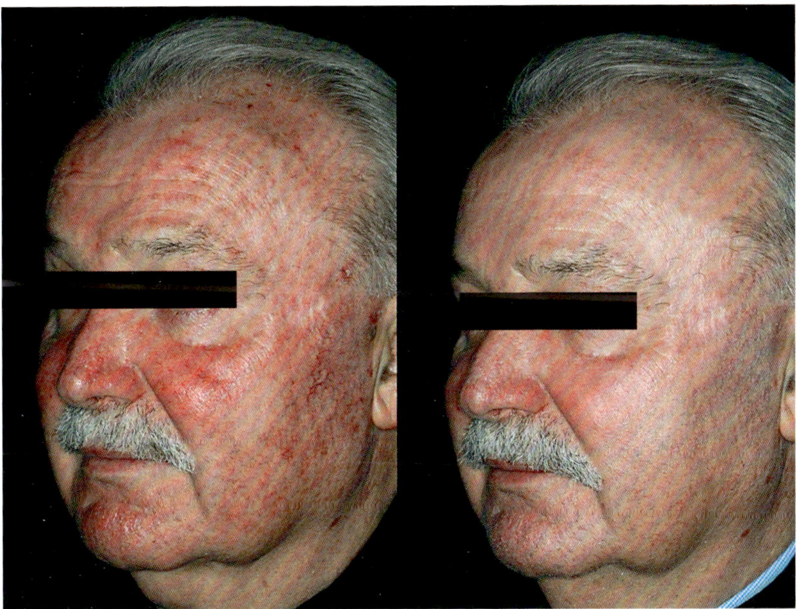

Fig. 10. Full face appearance of the patient of figure 9 before and after the procedure.

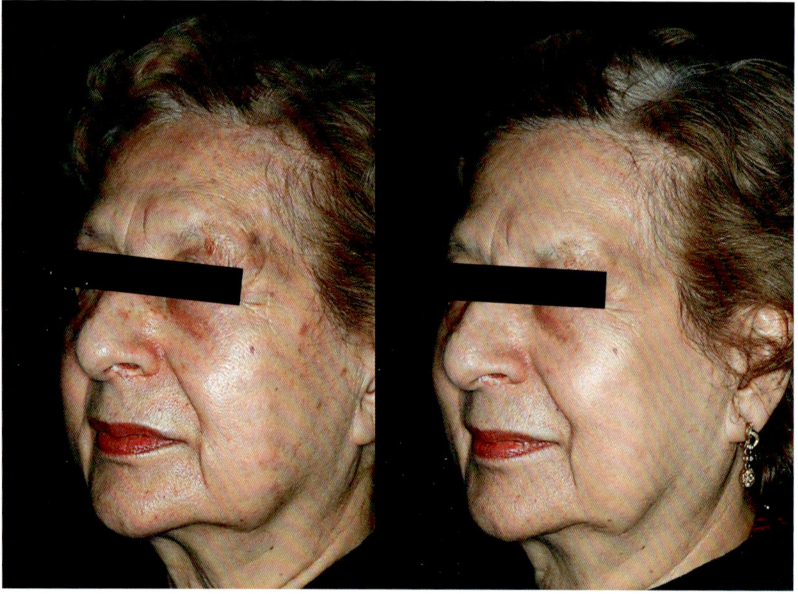

Fig. 11. 65-year-old woman before and 12 months after the procedure.

References

1 Gold MH: The evolving role of aminolevulinic acid hydrochloride with photodynamic therapy in photoaging. Cutis 2002;69(6 suppl):8–13.

2 Gold MH: Intense pulsed light therapy for photorejuvenation enhanced with 20% aminolevulinic acid photodynamic therapy. J Lasers Med Surg 2003; 15(suppl):47.

3 Goldman MP, Atkin D, Kincad S: PDT/ALA in the treatment of actinic damage: real world experience. J Lasers Med Surg 2002;14(suppl):24.

4 Avram DK, Goldman MP: Effectiveness and safety of ALA-IPL in treating actinic keratoses and photodamage. J Drugs Dermatol 2004;3(1 suppl):S36–S39.

5 Ruiz-Rodriguez R, Sanz-Sanchez T, Cordoba S: Photodynamic photorejuvenation. Dermatol Surg 2002; 28:742–744.

6 Alexiades-Armenakas MR, Geronemus RG: Laser-mediated photodynamic therapy of actinic keratoses. Arch Dermatol 2003;139:1313–1320.

7 Gilchrest BA, Blog FB, Szabo G: Effects of aging and chronic sun exposure on melanocytes in human skin. J Invest Dermatol 1979;73:141–143.

8 Green LJ, McCormick A, Weinstein GD: Photoaging and the skin. The effects of tretinoin. Dermatol Clin 1993;11:97–105.

9 Park MY, Sohn S, Lee ES, Kim YC: Photorejuvenation induced by 5-aminolevulinic acid photodynamic therapy in patients with actinic keratosis: a histologic analysis. J Am Acad Dermatol 2009;62:85–95.

10 Tschen EH, Wong DS, Pariser DM, Punlap FE, Houlihan A, Ferdon MB; Phase IV ALA-PDT Actinic Keratosis Study Group: Photodynamic therapy using aminolaevulinic acid for patients with nonhyperkeratotic actinic keratoses of the face and scalp: phase IV multicentre clinical trial with 12-month follow up. Br J Dermatol 2006;155:1262–1269.

11 Touma D, Yaar M, Whitehead S, Konnikov N, Gilchrest BA: A trial of short incubation, broad-area photodynamic therapy for facial actinic keratoses and diffuse photodamage. Arch Dermatol 2004;140:33–40.

12 Gold MH, Bradshaw VL, Boring MM, Bridges TM, Biron JA: Split-face comparison of photodynamic therapy with 5-aminolevulinic acid and intense pulsed light versus intense pulsed light alone for photodamage. Dermatol Surg 2006;32:795–801.

13 Marmur ES, Phelps R, Goldberg DJ: Ultrastructural changes seen after ALA-IPL photorejuvenation: a pilot study. J Cosmet Laser Ther 2005;7:21–24.

14 Orringer JS, Hammerberg C, Hamilton T, Johnson TM, Kang S, Sachs DL, Hamilton T, Fisher GJ: Molecular effects of photodynamic therapy for photoaging. Arch Dermatol 2008;144:1296–1302.

15 Dover JS, Bhatia AC, Stewart B, Arndt KA: Topical 5-aminolevulinic acid combined with intense pulsed light in the treatment of photoaging. Arch Dermatol 2005;141:1247–1252.
16 Wanitphakdeedecha R, Meeprathom W, Manuskiatti W: Efficacy and safety of 0.1% kinetin cream in the treatment of photoaging skin. Indian J Dermatol Venereol Leprol 2015;81:547.
17 Ruiz-Rodriguez R, López-Rodriguez L: Nonablative skin resurfacing: the role of PDT. J Drugs Dermatol 2006;5:756–762.
18 Babilas P, Travnik R, Werner A, Landthaler M, Szeimies RM: Split-face-study using two different light sources for topical PDT of actinic keratoses: non-inferiority of the LED system. J Dtsch Dermatol Ges 2008;6:25–32.
19 Gold MH, Bradshaw VL, Boring MM, Bridges TM, Biron JA: Split-face comparison of photodynamic therapy with 5-aminolevulinic acid and intense pulsed light versus intense pulsed light alone for photodamage. Dermatol Surg 2006;32:795–801.
20 Goldman MP: Photodynamic therapy; in Goldman MP (ed): Photodynamic Therapy (Procedures in Cosmetic Dermatology), ed 2. Philadelphia, Saunders, 2007.
21 Strasswimmer J, Grande DJ: Do pulsed lasers produce an effective photodynamic therapy response? Lasers Surg Med 2006;38:22–25.
22 Marcus SL, Houlihan A, Lundahl S, Ferdon ME: Does ambient light contribute to the therapeutic effects of topical photodynamic therapy (PDT) using aminolevulinic acid HCl (ALA)? Lasers Surg Med 2007;39:201–202.
23 Donnelly RF, Morrow DI, McCarron PA, David Woolfson AD, Morrisey A, Juzenas P, Juzeniene A, Iani V, Mccarthy HO: Microneedle arrays permit enhanced intradermal delivery of a preformed photosensitizer. Photochem Photobiol 2009;85:195–204.
24 Katz BE, Truong S, Maiwald DC, Frew KE, George D: Efficacy of microdermabrasion preceding ALA application in reducing the incubation time of ALA in laser PDT. J Drugs Dermatol 2007;6:140–142.
25 Fernandes D: Minimally invasive percutaneous collagen induction. Oral Maxillofac Surg Clin North Am 2005;17:51–63.
26 Fernandes D, Signorini M: Combating photoaging with percutaneous collagen induction. Clin Dermatol 2008;26:192–199.
27 Yoon J, Son T, Choi EH, Choi B, Nelson JS, Jung B: Enhancement of optical skin clearing efficacy using a microneedle roller. J Biomed Opt 2008;13:021103.
28 Henry S, McAllister DV, Allen MG, Prausnitz MR: Microfabricated microneedles: a novel approach to transdermal drug delivery. J Pharm Sci 1998;87:922–925.
29 Sklar LR1, Burnett CT, Waibel JS, Moy RL, Ozog DM: Laser assisted drug delivery: a review of an evolving technology. Lasers Surg Med 2014;46:249–262.
30 Sandberg C, Halldin CB, Ericson MB, Larko O, Krogstad AL, Wennberg AM: Bioavailability of aminolaevulinic acid and methylaminolaevulinate in basal cell carcinomas: a perfusion study using microdialysis in vivo. Br J Dermatol 2008;159:1170–1176.
31 Ruiz-Rodriguez R, López L, Candelas D, Zelickson B: Enhanced efficacy of photodynamic therapy after fractional resurfacing: fractional photodynamic rejuvenation. J Drugs Dermatol 2007;6:818–820.
32 Haak CS, Farinelli WA, Doukas AG, Tam J, Anderson RR, Haedersdal M: Fractional laser-assisted delivery of methyl aminolevulinate: impact of laser channel depth and incubation time. Lasers Surg Med 2012;44:787–795.
33 Haedersdal M, Sakamoto FH, William A, Farinelli WA, Doukas AG, Tam J, Anderson RR: Pretreatment with ablative fractional laser changes kinetics and biodistribution of topical 5-aminolevulinic acid (ALA) and methyl aminolevulinate (MAL). Lasers Surg Med 2014;46:462–469.
34 Jeffes WJ, McCullagh JL, Weinstein GD, Fergin PE, et al: Photodynamic therapy of actinic keratosis with topical 5-aminolaevulinic acid. Arch Dermatol 1997;133:727–732.
35 Babilas P, Travnik R, Werner A, Landthaler M, Szeimies RM: Split-face-study using two different light sources for topical PDT of actinic keratoses: non-inferiority of the LED system. J Dtsch Dermatol Ges 2008;6:25–32.
36 Peikert JM, Krywonis NA, Rest EB, Zachary CB: The efficacy of various degreasing agents used in trichloroacetic acid peels. J Dermatol Surg Oncol 1994;20:724–728.
37 Mikolajewska P, Donnelly RF, Garland MJ, et al: Microneedle pretreatment of human skin improves 5-aminolevulininc acid (ALA)- and 5-aminolevulinic acid methyl ester (MAL)-induced PpIX production for topical photodynamic therapy without increase in pain or erythema. Pharm Res 2010;27:2213–2220.
38 Lim HK, Jeong KH, Kim NI, Shin MK: Nonablative fractional laser as a tool to facilitate skin penetration of 5-aminolevulinic acid with minimal skin disruption: a preliminary study. Br J Dermatol 2014;170:1336–1340.
39 Willey A, Anderson RR, Sakamoto FH: Temperature-modulated photodynamic therapy for the treatment of actinic keratosis on the extremities: a pilot study. Dermatol Surg 2014;40:1094–1102.

40 Schmieder GJ, Huang EY, Jarratt M: A multicenter, randomized, vehicle-controlled phase 2 study of blue light photodynamic therapy with aminolevulinic acid HCl 20% topical solution for the treatment of actinic keratoses on the upper extremities: the effect of occlusion during the drug incubation period. J Drugs Dermatol 2012;11:1483–1489.

41 Wiegell SR, Stender IM, Na R, Wulf HC: Pain associated with photodynamic therapy using 5-aminolevulinic acid or 5-aminolevulinic acid methylester on tape-stripped normal skin. Arch Dermatol 2003;139: 1173–1177.

42 Garcia B, Goldman MP, Gold MH: Comparison of pre- and/or postphotodynamic therapy and intense pulsed light treatment protocols for the reduction of postprocedure-associated symptoms and enhancement of therapeutic efficacy. J Drugs Dermatol 2007; 6:924–928.

43 Clementoni MT, Roscher MB, Munavalli GS: Photodynamic photorejuvenation of the face with a combination of microneedling, red light, and broadband pulsed light. Lasers Surg Med 2010;42:150–159.

Girish S. Munavalli, MD, MHS, FACMS, FAAD
Dermatology, Laser, and Vein Specialists of the Carolinas, PLLC
1918 Randolph Road, Suite 550, Charlotte, NC 28207 (USA)
E-Mail gmunavalli@carolinaskin.com

Gold MH (ed): Cosmetic Photodynamic Therapy. Aesthet Dermatol. Basel, Karger, 2016, vol 3, pp 85–102
DOI: 10.1159/000439341

Photodynamic Therapy for Acne Vulgaris and Sebaceous Gland Hyperplasia

Amy Forman Taub[a, b] · Ann Cameron Schieber[a]

[a]Advanced Dermatology, Lincolnshire, Ill., and [b]Department of Dermatology, Northwestern University School of Medicine, Chicago, Ill., USA

Abstract

Photodynamic therapy (PDT) as a treatment for acne has been proven to be highly efficacious. The choice of the light source, photosensitizer type and dose, light source and dosimetry, incubation time and number of treatments and spacing makes protocols for PDT complicated. 5-Aminolevulinic acid, methyl aminolevulinic acid, methylene blue, indole acetic acid, and indocyanine green have all been used successfully as photosensitizing agents. Red light, pulsed dye lasers, intense pulsed light, and blue light have also been employed with good results. Complications can include discomfort, scaling, and sterile pustulation. Pain during procedures is not an issue for pulsed light devices; reducing the energy used for red light from that used for eradication of actinic keratosis mitigates the side effects. The mechanism of action is thought to include apoptosis of sebaceous glands (SGs), immune modulation, reduction in sebum secretion, and bactericidal effects. Although limited studies exist, PDT for treatment of SG hyperplasia has also been found to be effective. Calls for reduction in antibiotic use by the Centers for Disease Control, the President of the United States, and the thought leaders in acne mean that PDT should become a more commonly used treatment for acne. Limitations to its use include lack of commercial insurance coverage, need for avoidance of light for 48 h, and side effects. Enhancements to PDT may include heating and/or microdermabrasion prior to treatment. PDT continues to be one of the most effective treatments for inflammatory acne.

Introduction

Photodynamic therapy (PDT) for acne vulgaris has been an important alternative for patients who fail traditional therapy, or who cannot or choose not to tolerate systemic or topical therapies. Available now for over 10 years, there is significant literature of small studies showing effectiveness and safety of this therapy, as well as practitioners all over the world employing these methods to treat patients.

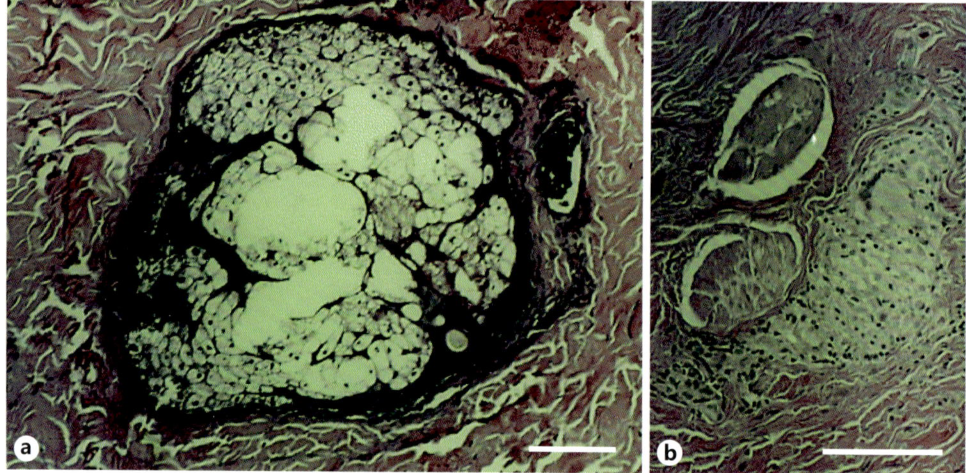

Fig. 1. Twenty weeks after 4 ALA-PDT treatments, there were atrophic or partially damaged SGs (**a**) and a granulomatous reaction in completely destroyed SGs (**b**). Bar = 100 µm [3].

Recent calls to limit antibiotics due to concerns over bacterial resistance [1] make this therapy ever more attractive. Barriers to usage remain economic and practical, in that the treatment is off-label and remains unreimbursed by commercial medical insurance. Also, treatment usually requires avoidance of sunlight for 48 h. Despite these drawbacks, use of this therapy continues to increase worldwide, and it is hoped that with better protocols the costs can be contained and the barriers overcome.

Sebaceous gland (SG) hyperplasia is a common occurrence, which appears to be associated with photodamage and age. Most treatments are local and destructive in nature, but usually only address the surface component, leading to rapid recurrence. PDT represents an alternative treatment that targets the deeper portion of the gland, potentially leading to longer-term resolution.

Mechanism of Action of Photodynamic Therapy for Acne

Although the efficacy of PDT in the treatment of acne has been established in clinical trials, the mechanism of action of PDT for acne is not firmly established. Changes in sebum excretion [2], damage to SGs [2, 3], *Propionibacterium acnes* levels [2], and immune system modulation [5] are all thought to be potential contributors.

Hongcharu et al. [3] suggested PDT (1) inhibits sebum secretion by injuring SGs (fig. 1), (2) sterilizes sebaceous follicles by killing *P. acnes*, and (3) reduces follicular obstruction by altering keratinocyte shedding and hyperkeratosis. Their demonstration of increased PpIX contained in SGs after application of 5-aminolevulinic acid (ALA) was heralded as the first breakthrough in explaining the mechanism of action. To date, there has not been an explanation for the differential uptake in SGs.

There is a high endogenous concentration of PpIX in the *P. acnes* bacteria that is not present in human keratinocytes. Since the absorption spectrum of *P. acnes* has peaks at 420 and 635 nm, blue or red light without additional exogenous photosensitizers has been shown to be effective for the treatment of acne [for PpIX absorption peaks, see chapter Gold, this volume, pp. 1–7]. This would most likely be a temporary phenomenon, since *P. acnes* usually recolonize within 1–3 months, making this a short-term therapy.

The addition of exogenous ALA may not make a significant difference for the destruction of *P. acnes* versus light alone. However, it has been demonstrated that PDT causes apoptosis of SG cells, a process that may take a few months. This may form the basis of the long-term effect of PDT on acne, versus the short-term effect of light alone. This may also explain why a 3-month follow-up after PDT yields better results than 1 month in some clinical trials [6]. Also, the destruction of the SG as the primary mechanism of action is supported by the fact that wavelengths of light that penetrate more deeply, e.g. intense pulsed light (IPL), pulsed dye laser (PDL), and red light, are more efficacious for acne treatment with PDT.

Another important component of PDT is the immunological effect of PDT. Jeong et al. [5] recently demonstrated that levels of Toll-like receptor (TLR)-2 and TLR-4 were markedly reduced in sebocytes. They performed PDT on 12 patients to assess its clinical efficacy and measure sebum secretion before and after treatment. The decrease in TLR-2 and TLR-4 expression by SGs and epidermis after PDT was 50 and 30%, respectively. In addition, TUNEL (deoxynucleotidyl transferase-mediated deoxyuridine triphosphate nick end-labeling) assays revealed increased apoptosis of SG cells after PDT (fig. 2). Increased IL-10 and decreased TGF-β_1 in fibroblasts after PDT may explain a reduction in inflammation and scarring, respectively [7].

Another method of attempting to localize material into the SG is to encapsulate it into a liposome [8]. These are structures that present a lipophilic face and hence penetrate more quickly into a lipophilic area, such as that of a sebum-rich follicular orifice, and have been utilized in formulated preparations of ALA.

Literature Review

Light Sources

The proper light source is critical for the success and minimization of side effects in PDT for acne. The light needs to reach the level of the SG, which is estimated to be about 1 mm below the epidermal surface.

Blue Light

Some portion of blue light reaches the level of the SG [9] as evidenced by the treatment of acne with blue light alone. However, the energy that is focused on the center of the SG may not be of sufficient magnitude to create the photochemical response needed

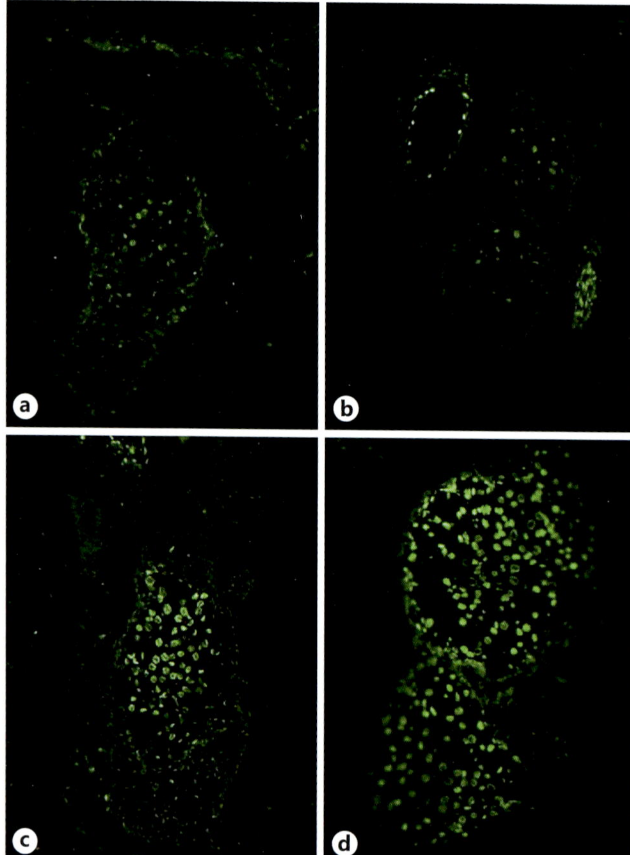

Fig. 2. Apoptotic sebocytes before (**a**, **b**) and after (**c**, **d**) PDT by TUNEL staining. ×400 [5].

to affect the gland cells themselves, as opposed to the bacteria around and within them. In a controlled study, Goldman and Boyce [10] showed that ALA-PDT with blue light was more effective against acne than blue light alone, and that short-contact ALA of only 15 min provided efficacy and minimal adverse effects. This was the first study to limit ALA incubation time to less than 1 h for PDT of acne. However, a later study found no statistical difference in the clearance of split-face lesions treated with blue light alone versus 10% ALA with blue light [11].

The latter findings are consistent with an unpublished disappointing study using Levulan and the BluU device for the treatment of acne. The study showed that the control side (Kerastick with vehicle only) performed as well as the active arm (Kerastick with ALA) for acne at 2 different doses, 5 and 10 J/cm^2. In fact, both arms irradiated with blue light showed a better improvement on the vehicle-only side than the ALA side. This result was baffling and remains unexplained. It also led, unfortunately, to the abandonment of further studies from industry regarding acne and PDT.

Red Light

Red light, on the other hand, appears to penetrate the SG quite well. It is used to treat basal cell carcinomas with PDT, and is estimated to penetrate the surface of the skin to approximately 1.5 mm. Unfortunately, red light has been associated with severe crusting, pustulation, and up to several weeks downtime [4]. More recent studies with lower incubation times have shown fewer side effects, although exfoliation is still common [12]. In a multicenter trial by Ma et al. [13], 397 patients were treated with grade II–IV acne with 3–4 sessions of 1-hour ALA incubation and 633-nm red light at 96–120 J/cm^2. The inflammatory and noninflammatory acne lesion counts gradually decreased after each treatment and during the 8-week follow-up. Maximum efficacy was obtained 8 weeks after the treatment completion.

The use of red light PDT for acne conglobata has recently been reported in the literature, given difficult curability and scar formation with traditional treatment methods. In a study by Yang et al. [14], 75 patients with facial acne conglobata received PDT with 5% ALA and red light once every 10 days for 1 month (n = 35) or a Chinese herbal medicine mask plus red light once per week (n = 40) for the same duration. Treatment with red light PDT significantly improved acne lesions and reduced scar formation compared to the control group. In addition, a study utilizing 10% ALA and red light demonstrated that PDT effectively reduces the area and density of macrocomedones utilizing a cyanoacrylate follicular biopsy [15].

Pulsed Dye Laser

PDL also employs wavelengths with the required depth to reach the SG. A randomized, controlled, split-face, single-blind study of 44 patients with facial acne sought to examine the efficacy of PDT using ALA and PDL [16]. Global acne severity ratings improved bilaterally with improvement significantly greater in treated than untreated skin. Thirty percent of patients were considered responders to this treatment with respect to improvement in their inflammatory lesion counts, while only 7% of patients responded in terms of noninflammatory lesion counts. In addition, Alexiades-Armenakas [17] showed that ALA-PDT with long-pulsed PDL activation was effective in a high percentage of patients against a variety of acne lesion types with minimal adverse effects (fig. 3).

Intense Pulsed Light

Gold et al. [18] were the first to use IPL for ALA-PDT for acne and demonstrated its effectiveness. Twenty patients were treated for moderate-to-severe facial acne weekly for 4 weeks with a 1-hour incubation of 20% ALA topical solution. The device used was a novel IPL and a heat source that emitted 430–1,100 nm radiation at 3–9 J/cm^2 fluence. Twelve weeks after the final treatment, there was a 72% clearance in the 12/15 patients that responded to treatment. Taub [19] confirmed the efficacy of short-contact (15–30 min of incubation) ALA for patients with moderate-to-severe refractory

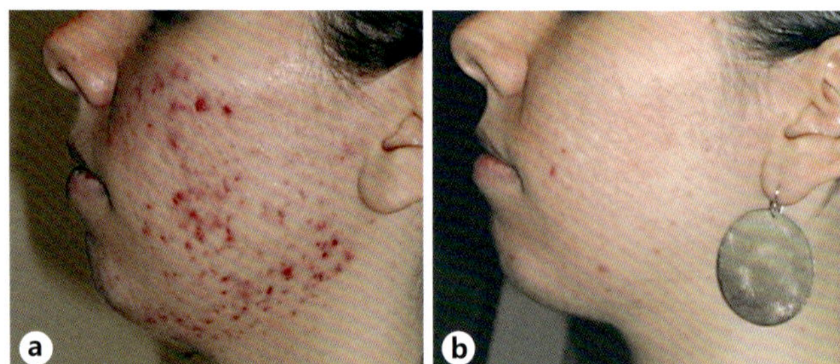

Fig. 3. Before (**a**) and after (**b**) ALA-PDT with long-PDL [17].

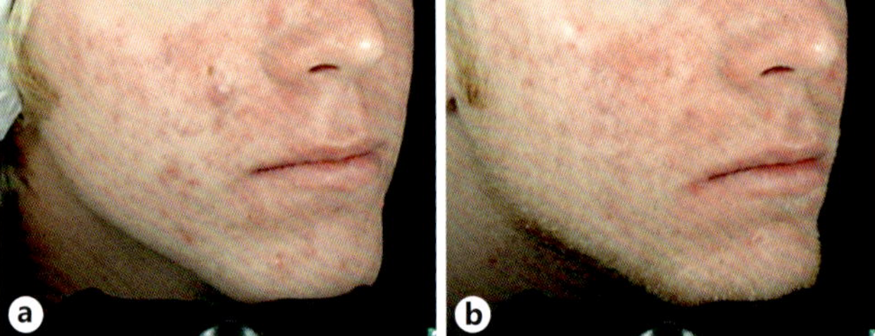

Fig. 4. Before (**a**) and after (**b**) 3 treatments of PDT with pulsed light with electro-optical synergy (photo courtesy of Amy Forman Taub).

acne. The results showed that electrical optical energy (IPL with bipolar radiofrequency) technology was an effective activator of ALA (fig. 4).

More recently, Mei et al. [20] demonstrated the efficacy and safety of ALA-PDT with 420–950 nm of IPL in Chinese patients with acne vulgaris. Forty-one patients with moderate-to-severe acne were randomly assigned to receive PDT with 10% ALA-IPL versus IPL alone with a 1-hour incubation period. The mean reductions in global lesion counts for PDT with ALA-IPL versus IPL were 75.2 and 51.0%, respectively, after 4 treatments.

Shaaban et al. [21] compared the efficacy and safety of PDT using intralesional ALA with IPL and IPL alone in the treatment of nodulocystic and inflammatory acne vulgaris on the face and back. All patients experienced a reduction in the number of acne lesions on both sides of the body, but the reduction was significantly more on the PDT side than IPL-only side. Recurrence of lesions was significantly more likely on the IPL-only side.

There is only one study publication on PDT for the treatment of SG hyperplasia. Patients received 4 monthly treatments of 15-min ALA incubation and IPL and had a 50% reduction in lesion number [56].

Summary and Conclusion

Given the plethora of lasers and data for PDT, Taub et al. [6] compared IPL, electrical optical energy, and blue light devices as activators in ALA-PDT. Acne grade and lesion count data showed 70, 60, and 30% improvement associated with activation by IPL, electrical optical energy, and blue light, respectively, 3 months after 3 monthly

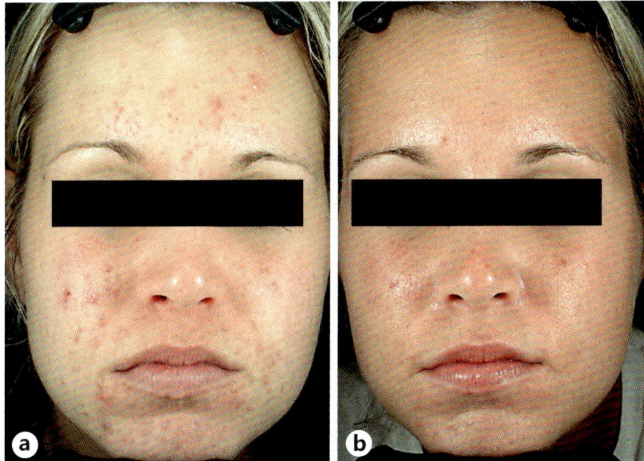

Fig. 5. Before (**a**) and 3 months after (**b**) 3 treatments with ALA and IPL (600–850 nm; photo courtesy of Amy Forman Taub).

treatments (fig. 5). The authors concluded IPL was the superior light source for acne (fig. 5).

In 2014, a meta-analysis identified 14 randomized, controlled trials involving 492 patients treated for acne with PDT [22]. Photosensitizers included ALA, methyl aminolevulinic acid (MAL), and indole-3-acetic acid (IAA). Light sources included red light, PDL, IPL, long-pulsed PDL, and green light. All treatments showed efficacy on inflammatory lesions, yet ALA combined with red light also had effects on noninflammatory lesions. Both PDL and IPL employ wavelengths with the requisite depth to reach the SG. It is possible that pulsed light, which features high peak power at short pulse durations, can lead to a pronounced effect with fewer side effects. The off-time between pulses may spare the epidermis; alternatively the intensity of continuous (red) light may explode the gland as opposed to inducing apoptosis, causing increased inflammation. Additional inflammatory material in the dermis might induce pustulation, crusting, and acne flares, for example. Although still effective to eradicate the SG, the side effects of continuous-wavelength light may make its use more fraught with complications. PDL and IPL are designed to have dynamic or surface cooling to reduce the overheating of the epidermis. The cooling may also be a factor in minimizing the reaction at the level of the epidermis as well as deeper in the gland. There are studies confirming that heat increases the amount of photodynamic reaction that occurs [23] whereas cooling inhibits it [24].

In conclusion, only light sources that can reach the SG (at least 1 mm below the epidermis) with high peak powers can induce SG demise. For ALA-PDT, those light sources include red light, IPL, and PDL. Pulsed lasers may be better than continuous-wave light due to their ability to achieve high peak power while avoiding overheating that allows gland contents to leak into the dermis, leading to excessive inflammation and side effects [25]. It is possible that lower photosensitizer doses and/or shorter incubation times might be able to achieve a better balance for red light with ALA/PDT [26].

Incubation Time

Investigators have invested significant effort to determine the effect of ALA dose, incubation time, and lesion type on PpIX production and treatment options. One study compared two different incubation times before performing PDT with IPL for acne vulgaris [27]. Three sessions of short incubation with ALA plus IPL (30 min, n = 9) or long incubation with ALA plus IPL (3 h, n = 11) on one side of the face and IPL alone on the other side were performed at 1-month intervals. All subjects showed improvement in inflammatory acne lesions, but the degree of improvement was greater with long than with short incubation or IPL alone. Similarly, Wang et al. [28] applied 10% ALA to inflammatory papules for 1–5 h followed by in situ fluorescence in order to examine the time course of PpIX production. PpIX reached a stable level after 3 h of incubation. Poisson regression analyses indicated lesion counts decreased by 0.791 times for a one-unit increase in incubation times (95% CI 0.782–0.799, $p < 0.0001$).

However, there are many studies showing efficacy of short incubation periods as well, as outlined above. The most important incubation time would be that which has a high efficacy for long-term clearance of acne lesions and is associated with tolerable side effects.

Identifying the factors that increase the ability of ALA to penetrate the SG and the kinetics of both its arrival in the SG and its manufacture of PpIX would be absolutely critical to improving the results of PDT for acne. The penetration of hair follicles by substances has different kinetics than that of a transepidermal pathway [29, 30]. This rapid diffusion pathway could be why very short incubation PDT can be effective in PDT for acne (fig. 6). Hair follicle absorption can take place in as little as 5–15 min whereas transcutaneous absorption usually takes at least 1 h. Of course, there are a huge number of factors influencing this: the size of the penetrating molecules, the lipophilicity of the substance, the temperature of the skin, and the thickness of the stratum corneum.

Dosage

To determine the effects of ALA dose and lesion type, Wang et al. [28] applied split-face 3, 5, and 10% ALA to acne lesions for 3 h followed by whole-face light irradiation at 633 nm and 30–70 J/cm^2. Similar PpIX levels were seen in areas receiving 3, 5, and 10% ALA. Poisson regression analyses indicated lesion counts decreased by only 0.999 times for a one-unit increase in ALA dose (95% CI 0.998–1.000, $p = 0.22$).

Kosaka et al. [31] showed prominent increases in PpIX 1 h after application of 5 and 20% ALA, while no increase was observed with 2.5% ALA until 2 h. A direct correlation was found between ALA concentration and ALA-PpIX fluorescence. While no fluorescence was detected 1 h after application of 2.5 or 5% ALA, 20% ALA produced strong fluorescence in the epidermis and SGs. Histological evaluation showed no damage to skin treated with 2.5% ALA-PDT incubated for 1 h, and damage was focused within the SGs with longer incubation times. Increased ALA concentrations resulted in prominent dam-

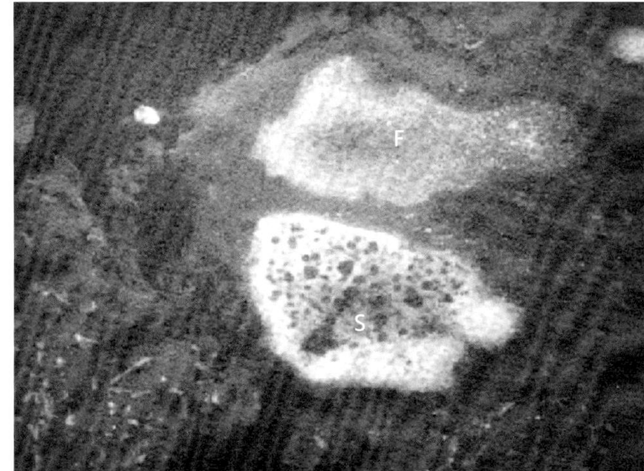

Fig. 6. PpIX production in SG: fluorescence microscopy shows PpIX production is greater in SGs (S) than in hair follicles (F) [3].

age to the epidermis and SGs, with deeper damage to the dermis when longer incubation times were used. Thus, PDT achieved improved safety and focused damage on SGs with low concentrations of ALA (2.5–5.0%) and medium incubation times (up to 2h).

Photosensitizers

The topical use of ALA in PDT was introduced and evaluated by Kennedy et al. [32]. As ALA penetrates epidermal cells, it enters the heme biosynthetic pathway (fig. 7) and is converted to PpIX, a photosensitive compound [11, 33]. ALA-induced PpIX is selective such that it only occurs in certain cells and tissues, and it has been found that strong PpIX fluorescence occurs in tumors or abnormalities that exist in the epidermis [33]. As ALA-induced PpIX accumulates in the epidermal cells, the ALA-treated area is irradiated with light, which, in the presence of molecular oxygen, activates PpIX to form singlet oxygen, an unstable intermediate that destroys the cells in which it is produced [34]. For photoactivation to occur, the light used in treatment must include wavelengths absorbed by PpIX.

PpIX also accumulates in pilosebaceous units [2]. In their 2000 landmark study, Hongcharu et al. [3] confirmed this finding (fig. 6). Of main interest in acne therapy is the localization of photosensitizer in the SG.

In the United States, 20% ALA is available in only one commercialized form, the Levulan Kerastick, a single-use system that contains the powder and the proprietary vehicle developed by DUSA Pharmaceuticals, Inc. (Wilmington, Mass., USA) for maximal absorption into the epidermis. The original study for the approval of Levulan for the treatment of actinic keratoses showed that maximal epidermal penetration takes place at 14–18 h. Thus, according to the package insert and FDA approval, the use of Levulan is for a 14- to 18-hour incubation (i.e. overnight) with the BluU device

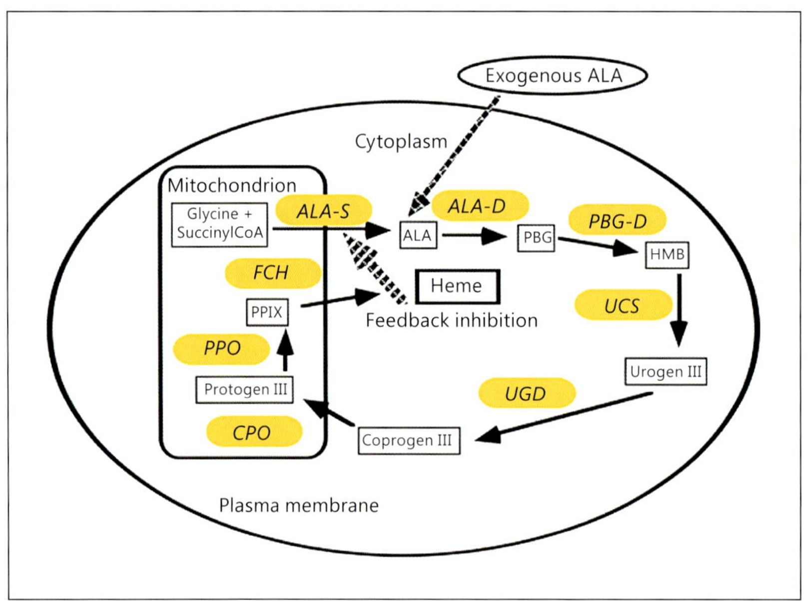

Fig. 7. Heme biosynthetic pathway [55, fig. 16]. *ALA-D* = ALA dehydratase; *ALA-S* = ALA synthetase; Coprogen III = coproporphyrinogen III; *CPO* = coproporphyrinogen oxidase; *FCH* = ferrochelatase; HMB = hydroxymethylbilane, *PBG-D* = porphobilinogen deaminase; protogen III = protoporphyrinogen; *PPO* = protoporphyrinogen oxidase; Urogen III = uroporphyrinogen III; *UCS* = uroporphyrinogen cosynthase, *UGD* = uroporphyrinogen decarboxylase.

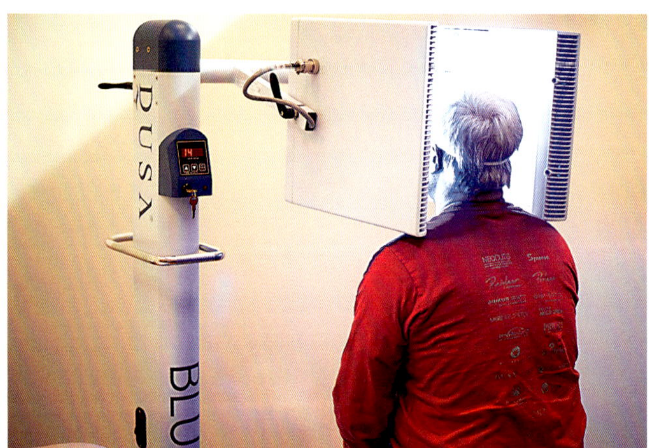

Fig. 8. Facial configuration of the BluU illuminator.

(415 nm; fig. 8) and usage for actinic keratoses only. The Kerastick with the BluU device for acne is an off-label usage.

A different commercially available photosensitizer, 16.8% MAL, is used primarily in Europe, Australia, New Zealand, Canada, and elsewhere. Approved by the FDA under the name Metvixia in 2008, the drug was not promoted by Galderma after a few years due to weak sales in the US. It is still widely used under the brand name Metvix in other countries. MAL is converted to ALA in the cell. Metvix is a cream rather than a hydroalcoholic solution like Levulan. There is some debate in the literature as to which is superior in terms of penetration and side effects. However, for the purposes of this chapter, this will not be evaluated closely. Both are valid forms of photosensitizer, but for acne the protocols would most likely differ. In an early study, 21 patients had 2 treatments with red light and MAL and exhibited a 68% clearance of inflammatory lesions [4]. Most patients exhibited significant crusting, erythema, and pustulation, 21 patients had MAL applied to their face for 3 h with one side receiving red light at 22 J (usual dosing being 37 J) and the other side receiving IPL at 8–10 J (also a reduced dose). Both showed effectiveness and no significant side effects [35]. Another recent study [12] used a 90-min incubation of MAL with occlusion and 37 J of red light using a Waldman® PDT 1200 lamp for acne vulgaris. Clearly, with MAL, as with ALA, there is also not a significant consensus on the best protocol.

Data on photosensitizers other than ALA and MAL have been published as effective agents in the reduction of acne. One is indocyanine green (ICG), a dye used primarily as a diagnostic aid for blood volume determination, cardiac output, and hepatic function. In 2002, ICG was first evaluated as a potential photosensitizer for acne when a study documented it was absorbed preferentially in the SG, which could lead to SG necrosis and acne reduction [17]. A recent study demonstrated the use of 0.6% topical ICG with a 30-min incubation period yielded beneficial results for the treatment of acne [36]. In both studies, a diode laser in the near-infrared range of 800 nm was utilized as this is recognized as the peak absorption of ICG (LightSheer; Lumenis, Yokneam, Israel). Although ICG is readily available in an injectable form, there is no established formula or commercial preparation in usage. As a result of this, Dr. Lloyd's group has ceased using this therapy for acne [pers. commun.]. One important advantage that ICG would have over ALA is the lack of absorption in the visible or UV range, making it unlikely that exposure to daylight would extend the period of photosensitivity, thus diminishing potential complications and making compliance with therapy easier.

Methylene blue is another photosensitizer shown to kill different types of bacteria and viruses [37]. This substance is utilized in humans for the treatment of methemoglobinemia, urolithiasis, and cyanide poisoning, and has been demonstrated to be nontoxic to human tissues for over 100 years [7, 38]. This photosensitizer is manufactured in a liposomal form and utilized for acne. In one study, investigators implemented a 15-min incubation period under occlusion and irradiated the treatment area with a red light diode laser for 2 treatments [39]. The data illustrated significant improvement in 2 acne grades after 12 weeks. Over 90% of the patients in the study showed improvement. The data also provide evidence that only the liposomal variant was exclusively taken up by the SG and not by other chromophores [39]. This increases specificity and decreases the potential for complications. There is also less downtime associated with the use of methylene blue because peak absorption is at 610 and 660 nm, which fall within the range of wavelengths that do not affect most other endogenous chromophores, ceasing the concern of continued activation after treatment as visible light is unlikely to activate the photosensitizer.

IAA has recently been introduced as a new photosensitizer for the treatment of acne. In one study, 25 patients with facial acne lesions were treated with IAA-PDT and green light, and results showed IAA-PDT was an effective and safe treatment for acne [40]. IAA produced free radicals with green light irradiation, and IAA loses its photosensitizing ability after exposure to certain amounts of light [41]. This implies IAA-PDT would not require photoprotection after the procedure. In addition, IAA-PDT requires only a short incubation period and the procedure is relatively painless in contrast to ALA-PDT [40].

A study by Jang et al. [42] compared the safety and efficacy of PDT using ICG and PDT using IAA for the treatment of mild-to-moderate acne. Patients were treated with IAA with green light (520 nm) on half of the face and with ICG with near-infrared radiation (805 nm) on the other half (n = 34). There were statistically significant reductions in lesion counts and there were no differences between the two treatment types. Both ICG-PDT and IAA-PDT showed better responses for inflammatory lesions than for noninflammatory lesions. The authors concluded both PDT with ICG and PDT with IAA are safe and effective for the treatment of mild-to-moderate acne.

It remains to be determined which photosensitizers are optimal for acne. ALA has an advantage in that it is commercially available and has a propensity to be absorbed by SG cells. MAL is also commercially available outside the US and has proven to be effective. Methylene blue, ICG, and IAA could be viable alternatives that might result in less toxicity following treatment. In order to optimize ALA as a photosensitizer for acne, it would be ideal to either perform a rapid treatment to avoid epidermal uptake and 'PDT effect', or to find something that could be applied topically or used systemically that could inactivate the remaining PpIX and thus the 48 h of light sensitivity.

In summary, the array of variables with PDT has proven to be a barrier to acceptance of this therapy. Clinicians are fearful of the severe side effects that have been reported with PDT, yet desire the best outcome for their patients. Balancing the incubation time, choice as well as dose of photosensitizer and light source has proven challenging. The literature has been somewhat contradictory as well. Studies have shown that longer incubation times are more effective, yet shorter incubation times can be effective. Lowering the dose of photosensitizer may be helpful, but they are not commercially available. Even choosing the light source is controversial, let alone whether dosimetry of light is an important factor.

Protocols for Photodynamic Therapy for Acne

PDT has been extensively studied in acne, yet without consensus on the optimal protocol. The US pioneers of ALA-PDT for acne formed the following recommendation for the treatment of acne [43]: Consensus panel members agreed that ALA-

PDT provides (1) the best results when used to treat inflammatory and cystic acne and (2) modest clearance when used to treat comedonal acne. They also agreed that (1) acneiform flares may occur after any treatment and (2) although not supported by extensive documentation, PDL activation provides the best results in ALA-PDT for acne. Thus, the American pioneers of ALA-PDT for acne formed an overall impression that IPL and PDL are superior light activators over blue light. It is prudent to mention that red light was not widely utilized in the US at that time.

In 2013, Morton et al. [44] published European guidelines for PDT. The authors concluded protocols employing lower drug concentrations, low light doses (e.g. 13 J/cm^2, 600–700 nm), short incubation, and less penetrating blue light are more likely to achieve a shorter effect via antimicrobial or immunomodulatory effects. In contrast, PDT utilizing higher energy (e.g. 150 J/cm^2, 550–700 nm) promotes direct destruction of SGs, and follicular obstruction may be reduced by enhanced epidermal turnover [45]. A recent analysis of PDT studies in acne concluded high-dose ALA- and MAL-PDT produce similar effects, photosensitizer incubation of 3 h or more was associated with long-term remission, red light is more likely to promote SG destruction compared with blue or pulsed light, and treatment was often painful and induced marked inflammation [46].

With these contradictory opinions, there are no clearly established protocols for PDT for acne, but certain common factors emerge when looking at published papers. Most American practitioners use 15- to 60-min incubation periods of commercially available 20% ALA (Levulan Kerastick). MAL (Metvixia), widely used in Europe and other parts of the world, is not currently available in the United States. Practitioner-designed formulations, such as ALA as cream or low-percentage liposomally encapsulated 5-ALA, have been used in Asia and Europe. Low-percentage liposomal ALA was designed to cause less side effects and to have better uptake into the skin, although it was used in a fashion where it was sprayed on the skin every 5 min for 60 min, negating some of the practical advantages possibly obtained by its use [8].

Pretreatment of the skin can be as simple as conventional acetone and/or alcohol degreasing of the skin or as complex as microdermabrasion. It is generally agreed that some preparation of the skin is necessary to allow the alcohol-based solution of ALA to maximally penetrate. Microdermabrasion definitely decreases the time for a PDT effect to be seen in the epidermis. In fact, microdermabrasion equalizes the erythema that ensues from a 10-min exposure to ALA versus a 1-hour exposure without microdermabrasion [47]. However, microdermabrasion, which ostensibly removes the stratum corneum (an important barrier to penetration) as well as some follicular occlusion of keratinaceous material, does increase the time and expense of performing the procedure. Common topical pretreatment options include salicylic acid preparations [48] or retinoids [49] although some practitioners avoid these for fear of exacerbated side effects. Nobody has done a study combining an automatic brush device

Table 1. PDT with ALA for acne: preferred and alternative protocols

PDT with ALA for acne	Preferred	Alternative
Incubation time, min	30–60	>60[1]
Light source	IPL, PDL, red	
Skin preparation	Acetone + alcohol	Microdermabrasion, heat, sonic cleansing
Interval/treatments, n	Every 3–4 weeks × 3–4	Every 2 weeks × 4
Maintenance	Every 2–6 months	

[1] May result in better sebocyte reduction but more side effects, thus limiting compliance.

for cleansing, which purportedly increases penetration of topical, following a cleansing session utilizing it [50].

Most commonly used protocols in the US are listed in table 1 with suggested enhancements.

Complications of Photodynamic Therapy for Acne and Sebaceous Gland Therapy

PDT complications are very well identified and understood. Pain with irradiation is often not present or rated very low during PDT for acne with pulsed light. Pain has been cited with red light and MAL [4]. Lack of pain can be explained by a number of factors, including short incubation times, use of pulsed light or laser instead of continuous light, reduced photodamage in younger patients, and the presence of the majority of the photosensitizer in the dermis as opposed to the epidermis. Short incubation times are selected for transfollicular absorption of ALA. This can occur extremely quickly, and the transformation of ALA to PpIX can likewise be a very fast process. If PpIX is then photobleached by the light source, there is little time left for ALA to be absorbed through the epidermis, limiting nonspecific activation. In addition, most people who seek treatment for acne are younger with less photodamage, resulting in lesser uptake by epidermal cells. Finally, with the reaction mainly taking place in the dermis, less surface change is usually noted. Even with MAL and red light, with reduced energy (22 vs. 37 J), efficacy was achieved without significant pain.

Another side effect is pustulation. Although secondary infection can occur, these eruptions are usually sterile and represent an explosion like a volcanic eruption. The sterile pustulation is caused by excessive SG inflammation. This is unsightly, uncomfortable, and limits compliance.

Peeling, blistering, and pain following treatment can also take place, especially if a patient exposes him- or herself to excessive light within 48 h of the treatment. This is one of the biggest practical barriers to PDT for acne. Although ALA or MAL is removed before treatment, a certain amount of ALA will continue to be metabolized to PpIX over 2 days, necessitating protection from UV light.

Strategies one could employ to avoid these dermal explosions yet still get a good clinical response and avoid direct epidermal exfoliation include reducing the concentration of photosensitizer, reducing the incubation time, changing the properties of the photosensitizer to make it more specific for gland uptake, using a light source that causes slower or more-modest fluorescence, or using a photosensitizer that is absorbed by a wavelength outside of the visible light spectrum [51].

Another possibility is that by heating the skin during incubation, the curve of PpIX generation can be shifted left [Willey A., pers. commun.], meaning that it is created more quickly and used up more completely. Thus, the need for protection from ultraviolet radiation may be reduced. This has not yet been proven but is a possibility that could advance this therapy.

Alternative Treatment for Acne and Sebaceous Gland Therapy

The Future

A new method of PDT with gold nanoparticles is being developed and will probably become commercially available in the near future [52]. With the laser treatment, gold nanoparticles are worked into the gland using an emulsion and a topical vibrating massage device. The particles are tuned to absorb near-infrared light, heat up, and cause thermal damage to the gland. The treatment uses 800-nm laser irradiation without anesthesia. Two studies were conducted on the laser therapy. In the first, 48 subjects were evaluated; 23 were treated with gold nanoparticles, and 25 used over-the-counter face wash (2% salicylic acid) for 12 weeks and then crossed over to gold nanoparticle treatment. At week 12, the mean reduction in inflammatory lesions was significantly better in the nanoparticle group than in the face wash group (34 vs. 16%, reapectively; $p = 0.02$). At week 16, the reduction in lesions was the same in the nanoparticle and the face wash/nanoparticle crossover groups (38 vs. 38%). At week 28, the mean reduction was larger in the nanoparticle group than in the crossover group (61 vs. 50%, respectively). Subjects reported mild-to-moderate pain during the laser procedure. Adverse effects included mild erythema, which went away 30–60 min after the procedure.

In the second study, the researcher team evaluated 49 subjects who received 3 treatments administered at 1-week intervals; 26 subjects received gold nanoparticle treatment and 23 received sham treatment. At 16 weeks, the mean reduction in inflammatory lesions was significantly better in the nanoparticle group than in the sham group (53 vs. 31%, respectively; $p = 0.045$). Published studies are in the works.

Another future possibility is the development of ALA either in a liposomal form or a heated form. Heating of the skin during incubation not only speeds and increases the metabolism of ALA to PpIX, but shifts the generation of the PpIX curve to the left, meaning that ALA is more completely photobleached (used up) with less of it around to become activated with light in the ensuing hours after the treatment has been completed. Standardizing therapy (perhaps with a handheld device of IPL) with heat and shorter incubation periods may also be a way of improving both the side effect profile and the overall results.

Finally, although not PDT, there are other potential treatments for acne that are energy based. It has been shown that the SG has an absorption spectrum that has peak wavelengths at 1,710 and 1,720 nm [53]. This has been shown to be clinically relevant in a study showing that usage of noncommercially available laser with a 1,720-nm wavelength was successful in eradicating SG hyperplasia [54].

Conclusions

PDT remains a very important and effective tool for the treatment of acne. With the mainstay of acne therapy being oral antibiotics and calls from the President of the United States, the Centers for Disease Control, and the acne thought leaders in dermatology for the reduction in their usage, the problems surrounding the best practice for PDT for acne will need to be resolved in the ensuing years and it should become a standard, commonly performed therapy for acne.

References

1 Dreno B, Thiboutot D, Gollnick H, et al: Antibiotic stewardship in dermatology: limiting antibiotic use in acne. Eur J Dermatol 2014;24:330–334.

2 Divaris DX, Kennedy JC, Pottier RH: Phototoxic damage to sebaceous glands and hair follicles of mice after systemic administration of 5-aminolevulinic acid correlates with localized protoporphyrin IX fluorescence. Am J Pathol 1990;136:891–897.

3 Hongcharu W, Taylor CR, Chang Y, et al: Topical ALA-photodynamic therapy for the treatment of acne vulgaris. J Invest Dermatol 2000;115:183–192.

4 Wiegell SR, Wulf HC: Photodynamic therapy of acne vulgaris using methyl aminolaevulinate: a blinded, randomized, controlled trial. Br J Dermatol 2006; 154:969–976.

5 Jeong E, Hong JW, Min JA, et al: Topical ALA-photodynamic therapy for acne can induce apoptosis of sebocytes and down-regulate their TLR-2 and TLR-4 expression. Ann Dermatol 2011;23:23–32.

6 Taub AF: A comparison of intense pulsed light, combination radiofrequency and intense pulsed light, and blue light in photodynamic therapy for acne vulgaris. J Drugs Dermatol 2007;6:1010–1016.

7 Byun JY, Lee GY, Choi HY, et al: The expressions of TGF-β(1) and IL-10 in cultured fibroblasts after ALA-IPL photodynamic treatment. Ann Dermatol 2011;23:19–22.

8 Yeung CK, Shek SY, Yu CS, et al: Liposome-encapsulated 0.5% 5-aminolevulinic acid with intense pulsed light for the treatment of inflammatory facial acne: a pilot study. Dermatol Surg 2011;37:450–459.

9 Ehrenberg B, Jori G, Moan J (eds): Photochemotherapy: Photodynamic Therapy and Other Modalities. Proceedings of SPIE, 1996, vol 2625.

10 Goldman MP, Boyce SM: A single-center study of aminolevulinic acid and 417 nm photodynamic therapy in the treatment of moderate to severe acne vulgaris. J Drugs Dermatol 2003;2:393–396.

11 Akaraphanth R, Kanjanawanitchkul W, Gritiyarangsan P: Efficacy of ALA-PDT vs blue light in the treatment of acne. Photodermatol Photoimmunol Photomed 2007;23:186–190.

12 Pinto C, Schafer F, Orellana JJ, et al: Efficacy of red light alone and methyl-aminolaevulinate-photodynamic therapy for the treatment of mild and moderate facial acne. Indian J Dermatol Venereol Leprol 2013;79:77–82.

13 Ma L, Xiang LH, Yu B, et al: Low-dose topical 5-aminolevulinic acid photodynamic therapy in the treatment of different severity of acne vulgaris. Photodiagnosis Photodyn Ther 2013;10:583–590.

14 Yang GL, Zhao M, Wang JM, et al: Short-term clinical effects of photodynamic therapy with topical 5-aminolevulinic acid for facial acne conglobata: an open, prospective, parallel-arm trial. Photodermatol Photoimmunol Photomed 2013;29:233–238.

15 Fabbrocini G, Cacciapuoti S, De Vita V, et al: The effect of aminolevulinic acid photodynamic therapy on microcomedones and macrocomedones. Dermatology 2009;219:322–328.

16 Orringer JS, Sachs DL, Bailey E, et al: Photodynamic therapy for acne vulgaris: a randomized, controlled, split-face clinical trial of topical aminolevulinic acid and pulsed dye laser therapy. J Cosmet Dermatol 2010;9:28–34.

17 Alexiades-Armenakas M: Long-pulsed dye laser-mediated photodynamic therapy combined with topical therapy for mild to severe comedonal, inflammatory, or cystic acne. J Drugs Dermatol 2006; 5:45–55.

18 Gold MH, Bradshaw VL, Boring MM, et al: The use of a novel intense pulsed light and heat source and ALA-PDT in the treatment of moderate to severe inflammatory acne vulgaris. J Drugs Dermatol 2004; 3(6 suppl):S15–S19.

19 Taub AF: Photodynamic therapy for the treatment of acne: a pilot study. J Drugs Dermatol 2004; 3(6 suppl):S10–S14.

20 Mei X, Shi W, Piao Y: Effectiveness of photodynamic therapy with topical 5-aminolevulinic acid and intense pulsed light in Chinese acne vulgaris patients. Photodermatol Photoimmunol Photomed 2013;29: 90–96.

21 Shaaban D, Abdel-Samad Z, El-Khalawany M: Photodynamic therapy with intralesional 5-aminolevulinic acid and intense pulsed light versus intense pulsed light alone in the treatment of acne vulgaris: a comparative study. Dermatol Ther 2012;25:86–91.

22 Zheng W, Wu Y, Xu X, et al: Evidence-based review of photodynamic therapy in the treatment of acne. Eur J Dermatol 2014;24:444–456.

23 Willey A, Anderson RR, Sakamoto FH: Temperature-modulated photodynamic therapy for the treatment of actinic keratosis on the extremities: a pilot study. Dermatol Surg 2014;40:1094–1102.

24 van den Akker JT, Boot K, Vernon DI, et al: Effect of elevating the skin temperature during topical ALA application on in vitro ALA penetration through mouse skin and in vivo PpIX production in human skin. Photochem Photobiol Sci 2004;3:263–267.

25 Lyte P, Sur R, Nigam A, Southall MD: Heat-killed *Propionibacterium acnes* is capable of inducing inflammatory responses in skin. Exp Dermatol 2009; 18:1070–1072.

26 Asayama-Kosaka S, Akilov OE, Kawana S: Photodynamic therapy with 5% δ-aminolevulinic acid is safe and effective treatment of acne vulgaris in Japanese patients. Laser Ther 2014;23:115–120.

27 Oh SH, Ryu DJ, Han EC, et al: A comparative study of topical 5-aminolevulinic acid incubation times in photodynamic therapy with intense pulsed light for the treatment of inflammatory acne. Dermatol Surg 2009;35:1918–1926.

28 Wang HW, Lv T, Zhang LL, et al: Prospective study of topical 5-aminolevulinic acid photodynamic therapy for the treatment of moderate to severe acne vulgaris in Chinese patients. J Cutan Med Surg 2012;16: 324–333.

29 Scheuplein RJ: Mechanism of percutaneous absorption. II. Transient diffusion and the relative importance of various routes of skin penetration. J Invest Dermatol 1967;48:79–88.

30 Kao J, Hall J, Helman G: In vitro percutaneous absorption in mouse skin: influence of skin appendages. Toxicol Appl Pharmacol 1988;94:93–103.

31 Kosaka S, Miyoshi N, Akilov OE, et al: Targeting of sebaceous glands by δ-aminolevulinic acid-based photodynamic therapy: an in vivo study. Lasers Surg Med 2011;43:376–381.

32 Kennedy J, Pottier RH, Pross D: Photodynamic therapy with endogenous protoporphyrin IX: basic principles and present clinical experience. J Photochem Photobiol B 1990;6:143–148.

33 Kennedy J, Pottier RH: Endogenous protoporphyrin IX, a clinically useful photosensitizer for photodynamic therapy. J Photochem Photobiol B 1992;14: 275–292.

34 Weishaupt K, Gomer CJ, Dougherty T: Identification of singlet oxygen as the cytotoxic agent in photoinactivation of a murine tumor. Cancer Res 1976; 7:2326–2329.

35 Hong JS, Jung JY, Yoon JY, Suh DH: Acne treatment by methyl aminolevulinate photodynamic therapy with red light vs. intense pulsed light. Int J Dermatol 2013;52:614–619.

36 Kim AR, Lee MS, Shin TS, et al: Phlorofucofuroeckol A inhibits the LPS-stimulated iNOS and COX-2 expressions in macrophages via inhibition of NF-κB, Akt, and p38 MAPK. Toxicol In Vitro 2011;25:1789–1795.

37 Morton CA, Szeimies RM, Sidoroff A, Braathen LR: European guidelines for topical photodynamic therapy. Part 1. Treatment delivery and current indications – actinic keratoses, Bowen's disease, basal cell carcinoma. J Eur Acad Dermatol Venereol 2013;27: 536–544.

38 Salah M, Samy N, Fadel M: Methylene blue mediated photodynamic therapy for resistant plaque psoriasis. J Drugs Dermatol 2009;8:42–49.

39 Fadel M, Salah M, Samy N, Mona S: Liposomal methylene blue hydrogel for selective photodynamic therapy of acne vulgaris. J Drugs Dermatol 2009;8: 983–990.
40 Huh SY, Na JI, Huh CH, Park KC: The effect of photodynamic therapy using indole-3-acetic acid and green light on acne vulgaris. Ann Dermatol 2012;24: 56–60.
41 Na JI, Kim SY, Kim JH, et al: Indole-3-acetic acid: a potential new photosensitizer for photodynamic therapy of acne vulgaris. Lasers Surg Med 2011;43: 200–205.
42 Jang MS, Doh KS, Kang JS, et al: A comparative split-face study of photodynamic therapy with indocyanine green and indole-3-acetic acid for the treatment of acne vulgaris. Br J Dermatol 2011;165:1095–1100.
43 Nestor MS, Gold MH, Kauvar AN, et al: The use of photodynamic therapy in dermatology: results of a consensus conference. J Drugs Dermatol 2006;5: 140–154.
44 Morton CA, Szeimies RM, Sidoroff A, Braathen LR: European guidelines for topical photodynamic therapy. Part 2. Emerging indications – field cancerization, photorejuvenation and inflammatory/infective dermatoses. J Eur Acad Dermatol Venereol 2013;27: 672–679.
45 Sakamoto FH, Lopes JD, Anderson RR: Photodynamic therapy for acne vulgaris: a critical review from basics to clinical practice. Part I. Acne vulgaris: when and why consider photodynamic therapy? J Am Acad Dermatol 2010;63:183–193; quiz 193–194.
46 Sakamoto FH, Torezan L, Anderson RR: Photodynamic therapy for acne vulgaris: a critical review from basics to clinical practice. Part II. Understanding parameters for acne treatment with photodynamic therapy. J Am Acad Dermatol 2010;63:195–211; quiz 211–212.
47 Katz BE, Truong S, Maiwald DC, et al: Efficacy of microdermabrasion preceding ALA application in reducing the incubation time of ALA in laser PDT. J Drugs Dermatol 2007;6:140–142.
48 Kleinpenning MM, Kanis JH, Smits T, et al: The effects of keratolytic pretreatment prior to fluorescence diagnosis and photodynamic therapy with aminolevulinic acid-induced porphyrins in psoriasis. J Dermatolog Treat 2010;21:245–251.
49 Galitzer BI: Effect of retinoid pretreatment on outcomes of patients treated by photodynamic therapy for actinic keratosis of the hand and forearm. J Drugs Dermatol 2011;10:1124–1132.
50 Akridge RE, Pilcher KA: Development of sonic technology for the daily cleansing of the skin. J Cosmet Dermatol 2006;5:181–183.
51 Taub AF: Commentary: how do we achieve consistent reproducible and clinically relevant results with PDT for acne? Dermatol Surg 2011;37:460–462.
52 Anderson R: 72nd Annual Meeting of the American Academy of Dermatology, Denver, 2014.
53 Sakamoto FH, Doukas AG, Farinelli WA, et al: Selective photothermolysis to target sebaceous glands: theoretical estimation of parameters and preliminary results using a free electron laser. Lasers Surg Med 2012;44:175–183.
54 Winstanley D, Blalock T, Houghton N, Ross EV: Treatment of sebaceous hyperplasia with a novel 1,720-nm laser. J Drugs Dermatol 2012;11:1323–1326.
55 Huang YY, Mroz P, Hamblin MR: Basic Photomedicine. http://www.photobiology.info/Photomed.html (accessed October 18, 2014).
56 Richey DF: Aminolevulinic acid photodynamic therapy for sebaceous gland hyperplasia. Dermatol Clin 2007;25:59–65.

Dr. Amy Taub
Advanced Dermatology
275 Parkway Drive
Lincolnshire, IL 60069 (USA)
E-Mail drtaub@advdermatology.com

Gold MH (ed): Cosmetic Photodynamic Therapy. Aesthet Dermatol. Basel, Karger, 2016, vol 3, pp 103–122
DOI: 10.1159/000439342

Chemoprevention Using Photodynamic Therapy with Aminolevulinic Acid

George Martin
Dr. George Martin Dermatology Associates, Kihei, Hawaii, USA

Abstract

There is global increase in the incidence of skin cancer. The associated morbidity and mortality associated with skin cancer has placed an increasing economic burden on health care systems. This burden has fostered an urgency to develop modalities to not only treat skin cancer and its precursor lesions, but also to provide chemoprevention to those potentially affected by this disease. Photodynamic therapy (PDT) offers a selective advantage over other modalities used for the treatment of a wide range of cutaneous neoplasms. Its ability to selectively, effectively, simultaneously, and noninvasively target and destroy a wide variety of skin lesions with little or no scarring make it an ideal therapeutic modality for treating cutaneous neoplasms. The commercial availability of standardized PDT over the last 15 years has led to a growing body of evidence on the safety and efficacy of PDT in treating cutaneous neoplasms such actinic keratoses and nonmelanoma skin cancers. Despite the numerous studies examining the therapeutic role of PDT in treating a variety of cutaneous neoplasms, relatively little evidence-based medicine exists to support the role of PDT in skin cancer chemoprevention. In this chapter, we will examine the clinical and scientific evidence for the role of PDT in skin cancer chemoprevention. Hopefully, the information provided in this chapter will provide direction for future large-scale studies that are necessary to further define the role of PDT in chemoprevention.

Introduction

Cancer chemoprevention has been defined as the use of natural, synthetic, or biologic chemical agents to reverse, suppress, or prevent carcinogenic progression to invasive cancer [1]. The global increase in the incidence of skin cancer in both men and women has resulted not only in significant morbidity and mortality of those affected but has also placed an increased economic burden on health care systems [2–16]. In countries such as the USA, Australia, Sweden, and the Netherlands where reliable records on the incidence of nonmelanoma skin cancers (NMSCs) are kept, younger patients are reported to be increasingly affected by NMSC [17]. However, recent reports from Australia show a decreased incidence of basal cell (BCCs) and squamous cell cancers (SCCs) of the skin in men and women younger than 45 years [5]. This decrease is likely due to nationwide skin cancer awareness and preventative measures developed in Australia.

Clinical research in the area of chemoprevention has focused on a wide array of therapeutic interventions targeting the initiating factors contributing to the development of skin cancer. A list of the potential therapeutic targets for skin cancer chemoprevention includes: ultraviolet (UV) damage [18], genetic mutations [19], viruses [20–22], and chemicals [23, 24] leading to tumor promotion and progression to carcinoma. Novel approaches [25–31] targeting these oncogenic molecular and cellular pathways include agents that have antioxidant, antimutagenic, anticarcinogenic, and immune-modulatory effects. Once cutaneous lesions have reached the carcinoma stage, the therapeutic focus shifts to targeted therapy of nascent lesions [30–32] and immune modulation [32, 33].

Photodynamic therapy (PDT) is an ideal therapeutic modality for skin cancer chemoprevention because it can target a wide range of diseases including skin cancer [34] while being safe and minimally invasive. PDT involves the topical or systemic use of a photosensitizer activated by a nonionizing wavelength of light that in the presence of oxygen triggers oxidative photodamage to selectively destroy targeted cells. From a historical perspective, the notion that PDT could target cutaneous tumors dates back to the early 1900s when von Tappeiner and colleagues first used PDT to treat tumors and diseases of the skin [35]. In 1984, Dougherty [36] reported on the use of an injectable systemic porphyrin photosensitizer known as Photofrin II, a derivative of hematoporphyrin. When injected, the porphyrin was retained in malignant tissue longer than in normal tissue and could be activated by visible light, particularly red light, to initiate a lethal phototoxic effect on tumors. It was the work of Kennedy et al. [37] that elucidated the mechanisms of action involved in topical PDT. Their work involved the use of topical 5-aminolevulinic acid (ALA) on abnormal epithelium to induce the selective accumulation of protoporphyrin IX (PpIX) that could be activated by visible light to perform PDT. PDT has evolved as a diagnostic and therapeutic modality for epithelial cancers of the skin, head and neck, esophagus, bladder, and lung [34, 38–41].

PDT has a therapeutic advantage over other modalities used in cutaneous oncology because it has the ability to simultaneously, selectively, and effectively treat a large number of cutaneous lesions over large surface areas with good cosmetic outcomes. Included in this spectrum of cutaneous malignant and premalignant conditions found to be responsive to PDT are actinic keratoses (AKs), NMSCs such as BCCs and SCCs, and certain cutaneous lymphomas [34, 42]. PDT also offers an alternative to surgical or destructive modalities associated with scarring, bleeding, or infection. These factors are important in managing patients with a large or continuous tumor burden who suffer from surgical fatigue or who are elderly. Because PDT is delivered in a clinic or hospital setting it avoids therapeutic compliance issues associated with self-administered topical or oral therapies.

Despite the many advantages of PDT as a therapeutic modality used in cutaneous oncology, there are little data available on its role in skin cancer chemoprevention. Large-scale well-controlled clinical studies providing long-term safety and efficacy data using PDT for skin cancer chemoprevention are lacking. To date, PDT studies have largely focused on its efficacy and safety of treating AKs and NMSCs but fail to prospectively examine the long-term role of PDT in chemoprevention. The lack of chemoprevention data is in large part due to the fact that PDT is relatively new to dermatology. Widespread access is a necessary step in gaining clinical experience using any modality and in particular for performing PDT. Prior to the commercial availability of topical ALA and methyl aminolevulinate (MAL) in early 2000, there was a lack of easy access to these standardized formulations and accompanying activating light sources. The majority of studies leading up to the commercial availability of ALA and MAL involved various dosing concentrations present in investigator-compounded formulas using a range of ALA and MAL dosing concentrations, which would then be activated by a variety of light sources using different protocols. Commercial availability and the accompanying standardization of PDT formulations and protocols led to the widespread use of PDT in dermatology.

Interestingly, despite the widespread availability of PDT and the accumulation of clinical studies examining its use in cutaneous oncology, there are scant available data regarding PDT chemoprevention of skin cancers. The data available on chemoprevention are largely derived from smaller-scale well-controlled studies in the organ transplant recipient (OTR) group [43–45]. Within the growing population of OTRs globally, a subgroup of OTRs has been found to be at higher risk for developing skin cancer because of the length of time and type of their immunosuppression, age at transplantation, 'fair' skin type (Fitzpatrick scale I and II), history of skin cancers, and cumulative UV exposure [44, 45]. This subgroup develops skin cancers, particularly NMSC, at a very rapid rate and is at high risk for developing metastatic disease. These 'high-risk' patients are most in need of a multidisciplinary approach to surveillance, therapeutic intervention, and chemoprevention. The therapeutic advantages of PDT in treating cutaneous lesions compared to other treatment modalities resulted in the adoption of PDT as a therapeutic cornerstone for these patients. From a clinical research perspective, the rate with which high-risk OTR patients develop skin cancers and AKs allows investigators to rapidly accumulate data pertaining to any therapeutic intervention or chemoprevention. Based on this reason alone, studies looking at chemoprevention in OTR patients require fewer numbers of patients who can be observed over shorter time spans in order to obtain meaningful data. Outcome data from studies involving the OTR group can then be loosely extrapolated to the nonimmunosuppressed population, particularly those who are at higher risk for developing skin cancer. Thus, much of the meaningful chemoprevention data on NMSC prevention reviewed in this chapter will involve studies in OTRs.

Chemoprevention of Actinic Keratoses

The largest body of clinical research involving PDT as a therapeutic and chemoprevention modality involves the role of PDT in treating AKs. AKs are neoplasms composed of highly atypical keratinocytes confined to the epidermis. They are considered part of the spectrum between photodamaged skin and invasive SCC [46]. This makes them an ideal target for chemoprevention studies examining the role of PDT in NMSC chemoprevention. The increasing worldwide prevalence of AKs among fair-skinned inhabitants in areas of high ambient sunlight is of concern [46]. The progression of AKs into invasive SCC on an annual basis has been estimated to range from 0.025 to 20% [47]. More recently, a direct observational study of high-risk but nonimmunosuppressed male patients was performed [48]. Individuals in the study were photographed and examined semiannually for the presence of AKs and skin cancer over a 6-year time period. The study reported the risk of progression of AKs into SCC (invasive SCC or SCC in situ) to be 0.60% at 1 year and 2.57% at 4 years. In their study, approximately 65% of all primary SCCs arose in lesions previously diagnosed as AKs. Further support for the ability of AKs to evolve into invasive SCC comes from a histological study of 459 SCCs of which 97% of SCCs diagnosed histopathologically were associated with AKs [49].

Scientific information linking AKs as a precursor to invasive SCC has resulted in the term actinic keratosis being used synonymously with 'precancerous' skin lesion [50]. Taking this association a step further, an increasing body of evidence involving clinical, histological, cytological, and molecular mutations supports the concept that AKs are de facto SCC in situ [50, 51]. This has resulted in proposed efforts to reclassify AKs using terms such as: 'keratinocytic intraepidermal neoplasms', SCC in situ, and SCC in situ *actinic type* [50–53]. Based on the consideration that AKs are noninvasive SCCs and because it is impossible to predict with certainty which AK will progress into invasive SCC, it is recommended that all AKs be treated [54]. For all the above reasons, it seems logical that PDT would be a necessary and ideal therapy targeting AKs in efforts aimed at NMSC chemoprevention.

The role of PDT as an integral therapeutic option for the treatment of AKs and NMSC chemoprevention has evolved over the last 15 years. This followed the commercial availability of ALA and MAL, their approved light sources, and well-defined treatment parameters [55–57]. Mechanistically, PDT takes advantage of the observation that the topical application of ALA or MAL results in the selective production of higher levels of porphyrins, particularly PpIX, in keratinocytes within AKs compared to normal skin [58, 59]. This selective accumulation of porphyrins is attributed to an altered cellular heme metabolism, which is most likely the result of lower iron levels resulting in the accumulation of the photosensitizer PpIX, the precursor to heme, as opposed to the nonphotosensitizing heme molecule. This is facilitated by abnormal stratum corneum overlying AKs, which allows for better penetration of topical ALA and MAL. The coupling of these two abnormalities in AKs enable topical application of either ALA or MAL to enter actinically damaged cells, bypass the tightly controlled rate-limiting enzyme ALA synthase, and result in the intracellular accumulation of PpIX and other porphyrins [58, 59]. The presence of PpIX in and around AKs allow for selective targeting with activating wavelengths of light when performing PDT.

There are several commercially available standardized drug/device combinations for performing topical PDT. In North America, a 20% ALA solution (Levulan® Kerastick®; DUSA Pharmaceuticals, Wilmington, Mass., USA) is approved for treatment of AKs of the face and scalp [60]. The approved activating light source and dose for the Levulan® Kerastick® is the BluU® therapeutic illuminator that delivers blue light (peak 417 ± 5 nm) at 10 J/cm^2 (DUSA Pharmaceuticals). In the US and Europe Union (EU), a 16.8% MAL cream [Metvixia Cream® (US approved); Metvix Cream® (EU approved); PhotoCure (ASA, Oslo, Norway)] is approved for the treatment of face and scalp AKs. Metvixia Cream®/Metvix Cream® is approved for use with the Aktilite® red light (610–650 nm; peak 630 nm; PhotoCure) [61]. Metvix Cream® is also approved in several European countries, New Zealand, and Australia for both superficial (sBCC) and nodular BCC (nBCC). In the EU, Metvix Cream® is approved for SCC in situ, also known as Bowen's disease (BD).

More recently, ALA and MAL have been compounded in various concentrations and incorporated into novel delivery vehicles including a patch. In the EU, a 4-cm^2 patch containing 2 mg/cm^2 ALA (total of 8 mg ALA; Alacare®; Spirig Pharma AG, Egerkingen, Switzerland) [62] and a gel formulation ALA (BF-200 ALA) with nanoemulsion of 78 mg/g ALA (Ameluz®; Spirit Healthcare Ltd. Oadby, UK) [63–66] used in combination with red light are commercially available. Both ALA and MAL are prodrugs which are metabolized in the skin to PpIX, the actual photosensitizer. Because PpIX has several absorption peaks in the visible light spectrum, the major one in the Soret band (400–410 nm, blue light) is the most efficient wavelength for activating PpIX, although longer wavelengths have deeper penetration into the dermis and thus maintain an advantage of treating deeper skin lesions [67]. In addition to blue and red light sources for PDT, other devices used to perform PDT include: pulsed dye laser (585 or 595 nm) and intense pulsed light sources (500–1,200 nm) [67]. Additionally, natural sunlight and ambient fluorescent lights are capable of performing PDT [67, 68].

When choosing a therapeutic modality for patients in whom chemoprevention is vitally important, safety and efficacy data using any of the available therapies require careful consideration and must be individualized. The available therapeutic interventions commercially available for the treatment of AKs in immunocompetent individuals recently underwent a network meta-analysis of their relative efficacy, which was published in a Cochrane review [69]. Included in the eight modalities studied were: ALA-PDT, cryotherapy, diclofenac 3% in 2.5% hyaluronic acid, 5-fluorouracil (5-FU) 0.5% or 5.0%, imiquimod 5%, ingenol mebutate 0.015–0.05%, MAL-PDT, and placebo/vehicle which included placebo PDT. Because comparator trials between therapies are lacking, in order to obtain a relative ranking of the efficacy of each therapy, the meta-analysis used as inclusion criteria: parallel-group studies for complete AK clearance and studies comparing at least two of the interventions. Based on calculated probabilities and odds ratios, the interventions were ranked as follows based on calculated probabilities and odds ratios: 5-FU > ALA-PDT ≈ imiquimod ≈ ingenol mebutate ≈ MAL-PDT > cryotherapy > diclofenac/hyaluronic acid > placebo. While several other factors are involved in the selection of a therapy for AKs in any individual, the review of available therapies provides a profile of relative efficacy in choosing any of the modalities. It also provides investigators evaluating chemoprevention therapies further insight into the comparative efficacy of potential modalities. Based on this review and others [70], it is clear that both ALA and MAL-PDT offer efficacy and safety profiles in treating AKs, which are equivalent or superior to other available AK field treatment therapies.

Specific information regarding treatment protocols, safety profiles, and efficacy data using ALA- and MAL-PDT to treat AKs can be gleaned from the pivotal phase III trials submitted to regulatory agencies for drug approval and discussed in the following paragraphs [55–57, 60, 61]. The protocols in these studies can serve as a starting point for any potential study involving PDT. It should be noted that the protocols involved in these pivotal studies were designed to maximize efficacy while maintaining safety. Study designs optimized lesion PpIX concentrations in face and scalp AKs following ALA and MAL application. Light exposure protocols were also optimized to provide maximum efficacy. However, these pivotal trials, which looked strictly only at AK clearance and not NMSC development in the treated area, provide little information on chemoprevention beyond the short-term AK efficacy data measured in the few months after treatment. Additional information on the ability of PDT to provide sustained field clearance of AKs (1 year) is provided by phase IV studies [66, 71]. Together, the pivotal phase III and IV studies on AK clearance provide valuable information and a starting point for chemoprevention strategies employing ALA- and MAL-PDT.

The approved protocol for ALA-PDT has evolved since it became commercially available in 2000 and is discussed in the following paragraphs. The approved protocol from the pivotal trials involves the application of a topical 20% ALA solution focally to AKs of the face and scalp followed by incubation overnight (14–18 h) [55, 60]. The overnight incubation was designed to maximize the amount of lesional PpIX and was based on fluorokinetic studies of PpIX accumulation following ALA application. This was followed by exposure to the BluU® light source for 1,000 s (10 J/cm^2). Lesion responses were evaluated 12 weeks following one or two treatments. For facial AKs, complete clearance was observed in 78% (108/138) of patients and for scalp AKs in 50% (21/42) of patients. AKs completely cleared in ≥75% of lesions: on the face in 92% (127/138) of patients and on the scalp in 74% (31/42) of patients. Data on sustained clearance were determined by a phase IV study [71] of 110 patients treated with one or two treatments with ALA-PDT for grade I and II AKs of the face and scalp. Complete clearance at 12 months was maintained in 78% of treated lesions that initially cleared.

The value of shortening the incubation times for ALA-PDT for practical purposes was evaluated in a series of investigator-initiated studies using shorter ALA incubation periods (1–3 h) [72, 73]. These studies were prompted by the inconvenience and potential hazard of inadvertent phototoxicity to patients when using 14- to 18-hour incubation periods. While less stringently controlled than larger commercially sponsored studies, they provided qualitative and to some degree quantitative data on the value of short (1–3 h) ALA incubation. In 2003, Smith et al. [72] demonstrated equivalent efficacy for a 1-hour ALA incubation followed by blue light PDT to a 4-week course of daily 0.5% 5-FU in providing ≥75 and 100% clearance. Touma et al. [73] compared full-face ALA application in 18 patients using 1-, 2-, or 3-hour incubation times followed by blue light at 10 J/cm^2. Clearance rates at 1 and 5 months were comparable to each other and to the standard 14–18 h of incubation.

Short-incubation ALA-PDT was recently evaluated in a large-scale commercially sponsored controlled phase II clinical trial [74]. ALA incubation times of 1 h (n = 47), 2 h (n = 48), and 3 h (n = 47) were studied on full faces, and a 2-hour incubation on a broad area of the face (n = 46) and followed by 10 J/cm^2 of blue light. Patients were evaluated for the percent change in AKs from baseline at weeks 8, 12, and 24. Following their initial ALA-PDT treatment, patients were evaluated at 8 weeks. Single-treatment individual lesion clearance results for 1-, 2-, and 3-hour, and broad-area ALA incubation were 35.7, 50.0, 56.3, and 57.1%, respectively. Patients not 100% cleared after a single treatment underwent a second treatment, which was conducted at week 8. Individual lesion clearance rates reported 4 weeks following the second treatment with the 1-, 2-, and 3-hour full-face, and 2-hour broad-area incubation were: 78.6, 76.5, 80.0, and 70.0%, respectively. Individual lesion clearance rates at 24 weeks for the 1-, 2-, and 3-hour, and broad-area ALA-PDT were 66.7, 64.9, 75.0, and 63.4%, respectively, but long-term clearance rates (at 1 year) are not available.

Based on this well-controlled study, it is apparent that a single treatment of ALA-PDT using short-term ALA incubation, while effective, is far less efficacious than ALA-PDT employing a 14- to 18-hour ALA incubation period. Two treatments 8 weeks apart provide a more substantial clearance rate that approximates the overnight incubation. This finding hopefully will guide future studies looking at the role of short-contact ALA-PDT in NMSC chemoprevention.

The pivotal trials [56, 57] substantiating the safety and efficacy of MAL-PDT for treating AKs involved focal application of a 16.8% MAL cream to AKs following curettage and occlusion of MAL for 3 h prior to its removal and illumination with a red light source. Two treatment sessions were administered 1 week apart. Multiple lesions may be treated during the same treatment session. Findings from Pariser et al. [56] using a noncoherent red light (570–670 nm; light dose 75 J/cm2) disclosed an 89% complete clearance of AKs at 3 months following two treatments in the treatment group (n = 42) compared to 38% in the placebo group (n = 38). Cosmesis was rated as good to excellent in more than 90% of patients. In a randomized controlled study, Szeimies et al. [57] compared MAL-PDT using a 3-hour application time followed by red light (noncoherent source 570–670 nm; total dose 75 J/cm2) to cryotherapy. Efficacy results from 193 patients with 699 lesions (92% face/scalp and 93% thin/moderately thick) were analyzed. Compared to cryotherapy, the overall complete (100%) response rate for MAL-PDT after 3 months was 69%, and it was 75% for cryotherapy. Responses were higher for thin lesions (MAL-PDT 75%, cryotherapy 80%).

Chemoprevention of Nonmelanoma Skin Cancer

Apalla et al. [75] published the first prospective study evaluating the effect of PDT on NMSC chemoprevention. They evaluated the hypothesis that field therapy using ALA-PDT could reduce the incidence of new NMSCs in immunocompetent patients with clinical and histological evidence of actinically damaged skin, i.e. field cancerization. They selected 45 patients with a prior history of NMSC in the area to be treated in a split-face study. Histologic confirmation of actinic damage adjacent to a confirmed NMSC in the treated area was obtained prior to the start of the study. These NMSCs included BCCs (16/45), SCCs (5/45), and AKs (45/45). It should be noted that AKs were considered histological NMSCs in the study as AKs were considered in situ *SCC* actinic type. The BCCs and SCCs were surgically excised, while AKs had received cryotherapy. Patients were randomized to receive a 20% compounded ALA cream to be applied to one side of the face and occluded versus placebo to the contralateral 50-cm^2 photodamaged skin on the face or scalp. This was followed by 3.5 h of light-impenetrable occlusion of both areas. The areas were then illuminated at a dose of 75 J/cm^2 and irradiance of 75 mW/cm^2 using a red light source (570–670 nm, Waldmann PDT1200; Waldmann-Medizintechnik, Villingen-Schwenningen, Germany). Two treatments 1 week apart were performed, and patients were evaluated every 3 months for 12 months for the presence of NMSC. Thirty-nine patients completed the study (30 males/9 females). The non-ALA-PDT-treated side demonstrated a linear increase in the number of new lesions over time. The treated side developed new AKs appearing at 6 months but overall had half as many new lesions as the nontreated side at 12 months (14 AKs vs. 30 new lesions: NMSC type unspecified). At 9 months, the rate of NMSC (inclusive of AKs) was equivalent to the placebo-controlled side. The chemopreventive ability of ALA-PDT to delay the onset of new NMSC lesions by at least 6 months was demonstrated. The ability of ALA PDT to reduce the occurrence of facial NMSC was evaluated before and after treatment with 5 sessions of ALA PDT activated by IPL. ALA PDT resulted in a reduction of facial NMSC from an average of 5 NMSC per year in the three years prior to ALA PDT to 1 NMSC per year in the subsequent year following treatment. This study suggests the potential for efficacy of ALA PDT activated by IPL may play a role in chemoprevention of facial NMSC [115].

Organ Transplant Recipients

OTRs represent a high-risk group of patients for the development of skin cancers and are a therapeutic and management challenge to both dermatologists and transplant specialists [44, 45]. A recent review summarizing the available data on skin cancer in solid

ORTs (SOTRs) provides valuable insight into the magnitude of the problem in these patients [44, 45]. NMSCs such as SCCs and BCCs account for 95% of skin cancers found in OTRs. However, SCC predominates over BCC, which is the opposite in immunocompetent patients with skin cancer. In OTRs, the risk of developing BCC is increased 10-fold, SCC 65-fold, SCC of the lip 20-fold, melanoma 3- to 4-fold and Kaposi's sarcoma 85-fold. SCCs, in particular, are more aggressive in OTRs, occur in sun-damaged areas of 'field cancerization' (i.e. extensive actinically damaged skin which may include BD), and have a higher risk of metastasis (8 vs. 0.5–5% in immunocompetent patients with SCC). Additionally, the number of SCCs developing in OTRs increases with time after transplantation. OTR data from both US and EU show that 10–27% of OTRs develop SCC 10 years after transplantation, which increases to 40–60% 20 years after transplantation. In Australia, 80% of OTRs develop SCC at 20 years.

The risk of an OTR developing SCC has been shown to increase with the presence of AKs, seborrheic keratoses, and warts compared to OTRs who do not have these lesions [44, 45]. Additionally, NMSCs usually develop in sun-damaged areas and particularly in areas of 'field cancerization'. In an attempt to lessen the morbidity and mortality caused by the burden of cutaneous tumors, a number of topical and systemic therapies have been studied. These therapies include not only ALA-PDT and MAL-PDT, but also topical 5-FU, imiquimod, diclofenac, and topical and systemic retinoids among others [45, 76–79]. In particular, ALA-PDT and MAL-PDT have been used in several studies evaluating their efficacy in reducing actinic damage and preventing NMSC [80–82]. While these studies, described below, evaluate smaller numbers of patients than a large-scale industry-supported pivotal trial, they do provide insight into the potential of PDT as a viable chemoprevention modality in reducing tumor burden in OTRs.

The ability of ALA-PDT and MAL-PDT to effectively and safely treat AKs in OTRs has been demonstrated in several studies. In a comparator study, MAL-PDT using red light was compared to topical 5% 5-FU in reducing epidermal dysplasia and clinically visible AKs [78]. Topical 5-FU has long been considered a standard of treatment for AKs in OTRs. The study evaluated 8 OTRs in a single-center, open-label, randomized, intrapatient comparative study using two cycles of MAL-PDT 1 week apart versus 5% 5-FU applied twice daily for 3 weeks. Clinical and histological clearance data were obtained 1, 3, and 6 months following treatment, and demonstrated complete clearance in 8/9 MAL-treated PDT patients versus 1/9 5-FU-treated patients. Patient satisfaction and cosmetic outcomes were judged by patients to be higher for MAL-PDT compared to 5-FU. The histological and clinical confirmation of MAL-PDT using red light in the clearance of AKs in this well-controlled comparator study provides substantial clinical and histological information regarding PDT as a safe and effective alternative to 5-FU not only for the treatment of AKs in OTRs but also for its potential use in long-term chemoprevention.

The safety and efficacy of MAL-PDT and ALA-PDT to treat AKs and BD (SCC in situ) in SOTRs were also evaluated in two separate clinical studies performed by Dragieva et al. [80, 81]. The first study evaluated 2 SOTRs and 20 controls with histologically confirmed AKs or BD [80]. In this open-label trial, patients received one or two consecutive treatments of PDT 1 week apart. Following mechanical (curettage) or chemical (salicylic acid) removal of hyperkeratotic lesions, a 20% ALA water-oil emulsion was used and incubated for 5 h under occlusion. The treatment area was then illuminated with 75 J/cm^2 of visible light delivered at 80 mW/cm^2 by a noncoherent light source (Waldmann PDT 1200) with an emission spectrum of 600–730 nm. Following one or two treatments, patients were evaluated at 4, 12 and 48 weeks for the presence of AKs. Complete clearance rates were 94, 89, and 72% for the immunocompetent group, and 86, 68, and 48% for the SOTR group, respectively. The complete clearance rates were comparable in both groups at 4 weeks, but at 12 and 48 weeks, the SOTR group had significantly lower complete clearance rates compared to controls ($p < 0.05$). The authors noted that SOTRs had a larger baseline number of hyperkeratotic lesions compared to the immunocompetent patients, and, despite mechanical and chemical debridement, the hyperkeratotic lesions appeared to have a higher recurrence rate. Lesions on the back of the hands also responded less favorably than other areas such as the face or scalp. Pain defined as moderate or severe was present in half of the patients in both groups, occurred during the first 5 min of illumination, declined thereafter, and was minimal following treatment. The pain was manageable with a cooling device and oral analgesia. The authors concluded that PDT is a safe and effective treatment for SOTRs with results comparable to immunocompetent patients. PDT also allows for the possibility of retreatment of large areas of actinic damage with a low risk of cutaneous infections in immunocompromised patients. This is particularly useful as there was a decline in response rates among SOTRs over time that suggested to the authors repeated PDT treatments are necessary to maintain clearance in SOTRs.

The second study by Dragieva et al. [81] involved 17 OTRs with a total number of 129 mild-to-moderate AKs. In this prospective, randomized, double-blind, placebo-controlled study, two lesional areas measuring 4 × 4 cm within a patient were randomized for two consecutive treatments of topical PDT 1 week apart using either MAL (160 mg/g) or a placebo cream, both used under occlusion for 3 h. Hyperkeratotic lesions were curetted prior to treatment. The treatment area was then illuminated with 75 J/cm^2 of visible light delivered at 80 mW/cm^2 by a noncoherent light source (Waldmann PDT 1200) with an emission spectrum of 600–730 nm. Patients were evaluated 4, 8, and 16 weeks after treatment for complete resolution and reduction in the number and size of AKs present within the treatment area. At 16 weeks, the MAL-treated areas demonstrated clinical clearance in 13 of 17 patients. A partial response was recorded in 3 patients. Only 1 patient and all of the placebo controls failed to demonstrate a response. All adverse events such as erythema, edema, and crusting were rated as mild to moderate, and the treatment was well tolerated. In this intrapatient study, the authors concluded that PDT in SOTRs is a safe and effective method for treating widespread areas of actinic damage and potentially reducing the incidence of SCC in this population.

Following these early series of articles on the role of PDT in NMSC chemoprevention in SOTRs, a number of studies examined the optimum strategy for treating patients. These studies focused on the development of new AKs as a primary endpoint and the development of NMSC arising out of AKs as a secondary endpoint. In an open, randomized, intrapatient, comparative, multicenter study of 81 transplant recipients, Wennberg et al. [83] used MAL-PDT to treat AKs. In the target areas, there were a total of 889 lesions (90% were defined as AKs) located within the observed 50-cm^2 areas on the face, scalp, neck, trunk, and extremities. PDT-treated lesions (n = 476) were treated twice (1 week apart), and at 3, 9, and 15 months for a total of five treatments using MAL cream (150 mg/g) applied for 3 h and activated by a noncoherent red light source (630 nm). Control lesions (n = 413) received cryotherapy at baseline, and 3, 9, and 15 months. Both MAL-PDT-treated and control areas received lesion-specific treatments (83% cryotherapy) at months 21 and 27. The results at 3 months showed a reduction in new lesions in the MAL-PDT group versus the control group (65 vs.103, respectively; p = 0.01). The decrease was mainly in AK lesions (43 vs. 80, respectively; a 46% reduction, p = 0.006). However, at 27 months, the effect was not significant (253 vs. 312; p = 0.06). Based on these findings, the investigators concluded that MAL-PDT may prevent new AKs in transplant patients and recommended further studies. Another point that may also be gleaned from this study of 'high-risk' OTRs is that the durability of response in high-risk OTRs is relatively short lived (<1 year), and continuing and sustained treatments are likely necessary. It also provides useful parameters for the study of nonimmunocompromised individuals who are at 'high risk' for NMSC.

The most compelling study to date examining the direct effect of PDT in NMSC chemoprevention in OTRs comes from Willey et al. [84]. They studied 12 high-risk OTRs who had a median occurrence per individual patient of 20.0 (15.0–24.0) histologically confirmed and treated SCC in situ and SCC in the 12-month period prior to the initiation of the study. They performed cyclic ALA-PDT at 4- to 8-week intervals over a 2-year period. The dose of immunosuppressive drugs in the OTRs remained stable throughout the study. They compared the incidence of SCC (in situ and invasive) to the year prior to initiation of cyclic PDT. Patients were treated with a 20% ALA solution under occlusion for 1 h and exposed to blue light (417 nm; BluU) for 1,000 s at 10 mW/cm^2. Hyperkeratotic lesions were removed by curettage and ALA applied to the area. The lesion count at 1 and 2 years was 4.0 (3.0–5.0) and 1.0 (0.0–2), respectively, for histologically confirmed and treated SCC. The percent reduction from baseline was 79% (95% confidence interval, CI 73.3–81.8%) and 95.0% (95% CI 87.5–100%) at 1 and 2 years, respectively.

Previously, De Graaf et al. [82] studied the effect of using one or two ALA-PDT treatments 6 months apart to reduce keratotic lesions and prevent SCC in OTRs. In an intrapatient study in 40 transplant patients, one or two treatments of ALA-PDT on one forearm and dorsal hand were performed with the other hand and forearm serving as control. Is should be noted that thicker lesions were not curetted. When patients were assessed at the 2-year follow-up, 15 SCCs had developed in the 9 PDT-treated arms and only 10 SCCs in the 9 control arms. The authors concluded that one or two treatments with ALA-PDT does not appear to prevent the development of new SCCs during the 2-year follow-up study period but may reduce the incidence of keratotic lesions.

When comparing the findings of both studies, it becomes readily apparent that significant differences in protocols can have a dramatic impact on the outcome of ALA-PDT as a chemoprevention measure. First, the frequency with which ALA-PDT was performed in the study by Willey et al. [84] was every 4–8 weeks as opposed to two treatments 6 months apart in the study by De Graff et al. [82]. Given the rapid rate at which certain high-risk OTRs develop SCCs, it appears that more frequent PDTs are needed to destroy either precursor or incipient SCC lesions. Secondly, the use of curettage prior to treating hyperkeratotic lesions with PDT is likely to provide a better result by permitting higher levels of drug penetration into the affected treatment area. Thus, more frequent use of ALA-PDT and field preparation of the treatment area are more likely to provide significant improvement in chemoprevention outcomes particularly in the case of OTRs.

Chemoprevention of Basal Cell Carcinomas

BCCs account for approximately 80% of NMSCs. In the US, where tumor registries do not include NMSCs, this percentage represents an estimated 1.6 million lesions [85]. Clinically and histologically, the three major BCC subtypes are: superficial, nodular and, grouped together based on histology, morpheaform, sclerosing, and infiltrative. Among those affected by BCC, there are certain high-risk groups such as Gorlin's syndrome also known as 'nevoid BCC syndrome' (NBCCS) who are susceptible to developing hundreds of BCC [86, 87]. There is a wide range of therapies for the treatment of BCC and these include: excision, Mohs surgery, curettage and electrodesiccation, PDT, radiation therapy, laser therapy, cryotherapy, topical imiquimod and 5-FU, as well as vismodegib (Erivedge®; Roche Pharmaceuticals, Basel, Switzerland), a hedgehog pathway inhibitor used to treat locally advanced and metastatic BCC [88]. Among these treatment options, based on an evidence-based review of treatment options for BCC [89], surgical excision still remains the gold standard for removal of BCC with Mohs micrographic surgery utilized for high-risk lesions. On the other hand, PDT, cryotherapy, topical imiquimod, and 5-FU are most appropriate for low-risk lesions such as small sBCC on the trunk and extremities.

The majority of PDT-related studies for the treatment of BCC are focused on establishing treatment protocols and obtaining accurate data on clearance rates for several subtypes of BCC [90–92]. Outside of the use of PDT to treat Gorlin's syndrome or NBCCS [86, 93–96], data supporting the role of PDT as a chemoprevention strategy for BCC is lacking. The effectiveness of PDT is based on many variables, including the type, thickness and the oxygenation status of the tumor; the photosensitizer used, its ability to penetrate the tumor and the duration of its application; the activating light source, the ability of its wavelength to penetrate the tumor, and the duration of exposure [88]. In addition to selectively targeting BCC tumor cells, PDT offers an immunologic benefit in treating local BCC tumors that can result in an enhanced systemic immune response to BCC cells [97].

Despite the many variables involved in effectively treating BCC, MAL-PDT has been approved for the treatment of sBCC and thin nBCC (thickness <2 mm) in the EU, New Zealand, and Australia [42]. Across the available studies using PDT for BCC, it has been generally found that sBCCs respond better to ALA-PDT and MAL-PDT than do nBCC [90–92]. Clearance rates using MAL-PDT following a single, initial treatment [98] or two treatments 7 days apart [99] followed by a repeat two-treatment cycle at 3 months if required resulted in a 9% recurrence rate at 1 year [99] and 22% clearance rate at 5 years [98]. Lesions >2 mm thick are often treated with PDT following lesion curettage [100]. In fact, a 10-year histology-controlled study of ALA-PDT combined with curettage found 22/24 (92%) of lesions cleared with the combination [101]. It should be noted that despite MAL being more lipophilic than ALA because of its ester side chain that allows for deeper skin penetration because of this property, studies found no statistical difference between MAL-PDT and ALA-PDT when treating nBCC [102].

The largest histologically controlled study with 5-year follow-up using ALA-PDT for the treatment of nBCC compared two PDT illuminations with a 1-hour interval after prior partial debulking versus surgical excision [103]. Patients (n = 151) with 171 histologically proven primary nBCC were randomized to ALA-PDT (n = 85) or surgical excision (n = 88) and followed for at least 5 years. Clinical recurrences were confirmed histologically. At 5 years, 23 tumors had recurred in the ALA-PDT group and 2 tumors in the surgical excision group. Cumulative recurrence probabilities 5 years after treatment were 30.7% (95% CI 21.5–42.6%) for ALA-PDT and 2.3% (95% CI 0.6–8.8%) for surgical excision ($p < 0.0001$). Of interest was that 2 tumors in the ALA-PDT group recurred 72 and 91 months after treatment. Cumulative probability of recurrence-free survival post-PDT was 65.0% (95% CI 51–76%) for nBCC measuring >0.7 mm in thickness and 94.4% (95% CI 67–99%, $p = 0.018$) for tumors ≤0.7 mm. Based on the depth of the BCC on initial biopsy confirmation, the authors concluded that PDT might be an alternative for inoperable patients with thin BCC (≤0.7 mm). Surgical excision remains the gold standard. They acknowledged that the tumor thickness measured on initial biopsy might differ from the thickness of the total lesion.

It is quite clear from a treatment efficacy standpoint that PDT is a useful treatment option for sBCC and thin low-risk BCC. However, it is a poor choice for higher-risk lesions such as thicker nBCCs, particularly those located in the H-zone of the face, and morpheaform/sclerosing/infiltrative BCCs [91, 92]. However in certain instances, such as large BCC or BCC located in the mid-face H-zone for which conventional therapy may be very difficult, MAL-PDT has been shown to be a reasonably effective modality with estimated sustained complete lesion responses of 78% with good-to-excellent cosmesis at 2 years [104]. For patients choosing PDT for these higher-risk lesions because of comorbidities that make surgery difficult or who wish to avoid surgery for cosmetic reasons, clinical monitoring is important. Thus, based on the safety, efficacy, and cosmetic outcome data involving PDT treatments of sBCC or thin BCCs as well as its effectiveness on more-difficult-to-treat BCC, it is apparent that PDT has a potential role in BCC chemoprevention in high-risk BCC patients.

The Gorlin syndrome/NBCCS, the result of a PATCH1 mutation, often results in the development of hundreds of BCCs in affected patients [86, 87, 96]. PDT has been identified as a very useful therapeutic option for those severely affected patients [86, 93]. Additionally PDT has demonstrated efficacy as a chemoprevention modality in these patients. In a study of 3 patients with NBCCS in whom BCCs and basal cell follicular hamartomas covered 12–25% of their body surfaces, ALA-PDT (1–3 treatments) was performed on areas up to 22% of their body surface [86]. The overall clearance was 85–98% with excellent cosmetic results. Responses to PDT were durable up to 6 years. According to the authors, the lack of appearance of BCC in the treated areas compared to untreated areas of the body may have been the result of destruction of subclinical lesions [105, 106] or possibly due to a local PDT-induced response [97].

A consensus paper on treatment guidelines for NBCCS has been recently published [93]. It identifies 9 relevant reports involving NBCCS treatments and provides an expert opinion in arriving at their recommendations. They found MAL-PDT safe and effective for the treatment of BCC in Gorlin's syndrome. For sBCC, all sizes can be treated. For nBCC, better efficacy can be achieved in thinner lesions (<2 mm thick), which can be assessed by optical coherence tomography, high-frequency ultrasound, or histopathology [107]. MAL-PDT should be performed according to labeling but can be adapted depending on the clinical assessment of the patient's needs. Multiple lesions and large areas may be treated during the same session as long as pain management is monitored. The use of PDT has been shown to increase patient satisfaction and reduce the need for painful and scarring surgical procedures in this group [96]. Most importantly, the chemopreventive aspects of PDT should not be underestimated for NBCCS [86, 96].

Chemoprevention of Squamous Cell Carcinomas

PDT is a safe and effective therapy for SCC in situ (BD) [108, 109]. The largest experience treating SCC in situ with PDT is with MAL-PDT. Clearance rates for SCC in situ 3 months following 1 or 2 cycles (2 treatments 7 days apart = 1 cycle) of MAL-PDT using red light range from 86 to 93% with sustained clearance at 24 months of 68–71% [108, 109]. For SCC in situ >3 cm in good healing sites, MAL-PDT using red light (630 nm/37 J/cm^2) resulted in a 96% clearance (22/23 lesions) at 3 months following 1 cycle (2 treatments 7 days apart). Recurrence of 3 lesions was noted at the 1-year follow-up, but cosmesis was rated good or excellent in 94% of patients [110]. Thus, MAL-PDT for SCC in situ appears to be a viable therapy even for larger lesions by providing good efficacy and good-to-excellent cosmesis. The role of PDT in chemoprevention of SCC in situ has to date not been evaluated in immunocompetent patients.

One study evaluated BD, microinvasive BD, and nodular invasive SCC treated using MAL-PDT [109]. Patients received 1 cycle (2 treatments 7 days apart) using MAL (160 mg/g cream), a 3-hour incubation followed by 37 J/cm^2 of red light (635 ± 18 nm LED light source). Results for all treated tumors showed 3- and 24-month clearance rates of 57 and 26%, respectively. The authors concluded that MAL-PDT is an effective treatment with good cosmesis for BD (Broders' scores I and II) and microinvasive SCC. In contrast, MAL-PDT should be avoided in patients with superficial SCCs with a microinvasive histological pattern and for nodular invasive lesions particularly if poorly differentiated keratinocytes are present (Broders' scores III and IV). Risk factors for recurrences are the degree of cellular atypia suggesting poorly differentiated keratinocytes are less sensitive to PDT. Based on the poor efficacy rates and metastatic potential, PDT cannot be recommended for superficial SCCs with a microinvasive histological pattern and for nodular invasive lesions.

In summary, studies evaluating the efficacy and safety of PDT for both SCC in situ (BD) and invasive SCC demonstrate good efficacy using MAL-PDT for SCC in situ but a high risk of recurrence in the case of more invasive SCC following MAL-PDT. Because the involved studies targeted individual lesions and did not involve wide-area field treatments, the role of MAL-PDT in chemoprevention in these patients cannot be determined. However, the efficacy of PDT in treating both AKs and SCC in situ (BD), which are precursor lesions to more invasive SCC, reinforce the importance of PDT as both a field therapy and chemopreventive intervention.

Chemoprevention of Cutaneous T-Cell Lymphomas

PDT has been used to treat mycosis fungoides (MF), an indolent form of cutaneous T-cell lymphoma [111]. MF often involves numerous scattered patches and plaques with the potential to cover wide areas of the skin. The ability of PDT to selectively target and treat MF lesions, and potentially prevent the development of new lesions, not only makes it an attractive therapeutic modality but may potentially provide a degree of chemoprevention. In case of tumor resistance to topical therapy, PDT provides an alternative to more aggressive and invasive approaches such as chemotherapy, radiotherapy, and photochemotherapy. Scattered small-scale studies and case reports reported on the success of PDT in treating plaque stage MF (stage I) [111]. Objective responses of 75% were observed in 29 patients with patch and plaques MF following monthly treatments for 6 months [112]. Weekly MAL-PDT using red light has also been shown to be effective in cases of MF resistant to topical steroids, psoralen-UVA or UVA1 phototherapies [113]. However, case reports of recurrences months after cessation of treatment have been reported [114]. PDT is also limited to stage I disease, having decreased efficacy in treating the tumor stage of MF (stage II) [112]. While it appears that PDT is an effective adjunctive therapy for the treatment of stage I MF, treatment parameters for MF have yet to be defined. Furthermore, no studies to date have examined the chemopreventive effects of PDT on MF.

Conclusion

PDT has been extensively and effectively used for the treatment of AKs and NMSCs. Despite its potential as a chemoprevention modality, little compelling data regarding the effectiveness of PDT as a chemoprevention modality in immune-competent individuals is available. The effectiveness of PDT as a chemoprevention modality in high-risk immunocompromised patients and Gorlin's syndrome/NBCCS provides insight into its potential. Moving forward, large-scale industry- or government-sponsored studies are needed to validate the role of PDT in chemoprevention.

References

1 Tsao A, Kim E, Hong W: Chemoprevention of cancer. CA Cancer J Clin 2004;54:150–180.
2 Diepgen TL, Mahler V: The epidemiology of skin cancer. Br J Dermatol 2002;146(suppl 61):1–6.
3 Hemminki K, Zhang H, Czene K: Time trends and familial risks in squamous cell carcinoma of the skin. Arch Dermatol 2003;139:885–889.
4 Lebwohl M: Actinic keratosis: epidemiology and progression to squamous cell carcinoma. Br J Dermatol 2003;149(suppl 66).31–33.
5 Olsen CM, Williams PF, Whiteman DC: Turning the tide? Changes in treatment rates for keratinocytic cancers in Australia 2000 through 2011. J Am Acad Dermatol 2014;71:21.e1–26.e1.
6 Araki K, Nagano T, Ueda M, Washio F, Watanabe S, Yamaguchi N, Ichihashi M: Incidence of skin cancers and precancerous lesions in Japanese – risk factors and prevention. J Epidemiol 1999;9(6 suppl): S14–S21.
7 Eisemann N, Waldmann A, Geller A, Weinstock M, Volkmer B, et al: Non-melanoma skin cancer incidence and impact of skin cancer screening on incidence. J Invest Dermatol 2014;134:43–50.
8 Tejaswi M, Pearce D, Yentzer B, Williford P, Feldman S: The economic impact of non-melanoma skin cancer: a review. J Natl Compr Canc Netw 2010;8: 888–896.
9 The Economic Burden of Skin Cancer in Canada: Current and Projected. Canadian Partnership against Cancer, 2010, http://www.cancercare.ns.ca/site-cc/media/cancercare/Economic%20Burden%20of%20Skin%20Cancer%20in%20Canada%20Report.pdf.
10 Aguilar-Bernier M, González-Carrascosa M, Padilla-España L, Rivas-Ruiz F, Jiménez-Puente A, de Troya-Martín M: Five-year economic evaluation of non-melanoma skin cancer surgery at the Costa del Sol Hospital (2006–2010). J Eur Acad Dermatol Venereol 2014;28:320–326.
11 Fransen M, Karahalios A, Sharma N, English DR, Giles GG, Sinclair RD: Non-melanaoma skin cancer in Australia. Med J Aust 2012;197:565–568.
12 Health System Expenditure on Cancer and Other Neoplasms in Australia 2008–09. Canberra, Australian Institute of Health and Welfare, 2013, Cancer Ser 81.
13 Skin Cancer Incidence Statistics. Cancer Research UK, http://www.cancerresearchuk.org/health-professional/cancer-statistics/statistics-by-cancer-type/skin-cancer/incidence.
14 Lomas A, Leonardi-Bee J, Bath-Hextall F: A systematic review of worldwide incidence of nonmelanoma skin cancer. Br J Dermatol 2012;166:1069–1080.
15 Warino L, Tusa M, Camacho F, Teuschler H, Fleischer AB Jr, Feldman SR: Frequency and cost of actinic keratosis treatment. Dermatol Surg 2006;32: 1045–1049.
16 Bickers DR, Lim HW, Margolis D, et al: The burden of skin diseases: 2004 a joint project of the American Academy of Dermatology Association and the Society for Investigative Dermatology. J Am Acad Dermatol 2006;55:490–500.
17 Christenson LJ, Borrowman TA, Vachon CM, Tollefson MM, Otley CC, Weaver AL, Roenigk RK: Incidence of basal cell and squamous cell carcinomas in a population younger than 40 years. JAMA 2005; 294:681–690.

18 Mancebo SE, Wang SQ: Skin cancer: role of ultraviolet radiation in carcinogenesis. Rev Environ Health 2014;29:265–273.

19 Reichrath J, Rass K: Ultraviolet damage, DNA repair and vitamin D in nonmelanoma skin cancer and in malignant melanoma: an update. Adv Exp Med Biol 2014;810:208–233.

20 Smola S: Human papillomaviruses and skin cancer. Adv Exp Med Biol 2014;810:192–207.

21 Stakaityte G, Wood JJ, Knight L, Abdul-Sada H, Adzahar N, et al: Merkel cell polyomavirus: molecular insights into the most recently discovered human tumour virus. Cancers (Basel) 2014;6:1267–1297.

22 Molho-Pessach V, Lotem M: Viral carcinogenesis in skin cancer. Curr Probl Dermatol 2007;35:39–51.

23 Boffetta P, Jourenkova N, Gustavsson P: Cancer risk from occupational and environmental exposure to polycyclic aromatic hydrocarbons. Cancer Causes Control 1997;8:444–472.

24 Surdu S, Fitzgerald E, Bloom M, Carpenter D, Haase R, et al: Occupational exposure to arsenic and risk of nonmelanoma skin cancer in a multinational European study. Int J Cancer 2013;133:2182–2191.

25 Chen A, Halliday G, Damian D: Non-melanoma skin cancer: carcinogenesis and chemoprevention. Pathology 2013;45:331–341.

26 Singh M, Suman S, Shukla Y: New enlightenment of skin cancer chemoprevention through phytochemicals: in vitro and in vivo studies and the underlying mechanisms. Biomed Res Int 2014;2014:243452.

27 Nichols JA, Katiyar SK: Skin photoprotection by natural polyphenols: anti-inflammatory, antioxidant and DNA repair mechanisms. Arch Dermatol Res 2010;302:71–83.

28 Wright T, Spencer J, Flowers F: Chemoprevention of nonmelanoma skin cancer. J Am Acad Dermatol 2006;54:933–946; quiz 947–950.

29 Camp WL, Turnham JW, Athar M, Elmets CA: New agents for prevention of ultraviolet-induced nonmelanoma skin cancer. Semin Cutan Med Surg 2011; 30:6–13.

30 Walls B, Jordan L, Diaz L, Miller R: Targeted therapy for cutaneous oncology: a review of novel treatment options for non-melanoma skin cancer. Part I. J Drugs Dermatol 2014;13:947–952.

31 Walls B, Jordan L, Diaz L, Miller R: Targeted therapy for cutaneous oncology: a review of novel treatment options for non-melanoma skin cancer. Part II. J Drugs Dermatol 2014;13:955–958.

32 Vogt T: Therapy of metastatic malignant melanoma: on the way to individualized disease control. Adv Exp Med Biol 2014;810:272–281.

33 Rangwalaa S, Tsaib K: Roles of the immune system in skin cancer. Br J Dermatol 2011;165:953–965.

34 Gold MH: Photodynamic Therapy in Dermatology. New York, Springer, 2011.

35 Moan J, Peng Q: An outline of the history of PDT. Anticancer Res 2003;23:3591–3600.

36 Dougherty TJ: Photodynamic therapy (PDT) of malignant tumors. Crit Rev Oncol Hematol 1984;2:83–116.

37 Kennedy JC, Pottier RH, Pross DC: Photodynamic therapy with endogenous protoporphyrin IX: basic principles and present clinical experience. J Photochem Photobiol B 1990;6:143–148.

38 Nelke K, Pawlak W, Leszczyszyn J, Gerber H: Photodynamic therapy in head and neck cancer. Postepy Hig Med Dosw (Online) 2014;68:119–128.

39 Shishkova N, Kuznetsova O, Berezov T: Photodynamic therapy in gastroenterology. J Gastrointest Cancer 2013;44:251–259.

40 Darlenski R, Fluhr J: Photodynamic therapy in dermatology: past, present, and future. J Biomed Opt 2013;18:061208.

41 Allison R: Photodynamic therapy: oncologic horizons. Future Oncol 2014;10:123–124.

42 Ross K, Cherpelis B, Lien M, Fenske N: Spotlighting the role of photodynamic therapy in cutaneous malignancy: an update and expansion. Dermatol Surg 2013;39:1733–1744.

43 Brin L, Zubair A, Brewer J: Optimal management of skin cancer in immunosuppressed patients. Am J Clin Dermatol 2014;15:339–356.

44 O'Reilly Zwald F, Brown M: Skin cancer in solid organ transplant recipients: advances in therapy and management. Part I. Epidemiology of skin cancer in solid organ transplant recipients. J Am Acad Dermatol 2011;65:253–261.

45 O'Reilly Zwald F, Brown M: Skin cancer in solid organ transplant recipients: advances in therapy and management. Part II. Management of skin cancer in solid organ transplant recipients. J Am Acad Dermatol 2011;65:263–279.

46 Gilchrest BA, Martin G: Pitfalls of evidence-based medicine: the example of actinic keratosis therapy. Arch Dermatol 2012;148:528–530.

47 Quaedvlieg PJ, Tirsi E, Thissen MR, Krekels GA: Actinic keratosis: how to differentiate the good from the bad ones? Eur J Dermatol 2006;16:335–339.

48 Criscione VD, Weinstock MA, Naylor MF, Luque C, Eide MJ, Bingham SF: Actinic keratoses: natural history and risk of malignant transformation in the Veterans Affairs Topical Tretinoin Chemoprevention Trial. Cancer 2009;115:2523–2530.

49 Hurwitz RM, Monger LE: Solar keratosis: an evolving squamous cell carcinoma. Benign or malignant? Dermatol Surg 1995;21:184.

50 Ackerman AB, Mones JM: Solar (actinic) keratosis is squamous cell carcinoma. Br J Dermatol 2006;155: 9–22.

51 Rowert-Huber J, Patel MJ, Forschner T, et al: Actinic keratosis is an early in situ squamous cell carcinoma: a proposal for reclassification. Br J Dermatol 2007;156(suppl 3):8–12.
52 Werner RN, Stockfleth E, Connolly SM, Correia O, Erdmann R, Foley P, Gupta AK, Jacobs A, Kerl H, Lim HW, Martin G, Paquet M, Pariser DM, Rosumeck S, Röwert Huber HJ, Sahota A, Sangueza OP, Shumack S, Sporbeck B, Swanson NA, Torezan L, Nast A: Evidence- and consensus-based (S3) Guidelines for the Treatment of Actinic Keratosis – International League of Dermatological Societies in cooperation with the European Dermatology Forum - Short version. J Eur Acad Dermatol Venereol 2015;29: 2069–2079.
53 Cockerell CJ, Wharton JR: New histopathological classification of actinic keratosis (incipient intraepidermal squamous cell carcinoma). J Drugs Dermatol 2005;4:462–467.
54 Moy R: Clinical presentation of actinic keratoses and squamous cell carcinoma. J Am Acad Dermatol 2000;42:S8–S10.
55 Piacquadio DJ, Chen DM, Farber HF, Fowler JF Jr, Glazer SD, Goodman JJ, Hruza LL, Jeffes EW, Ling MR, Phillips TJ, Rallis TM, Scher RK, Taylor CR, Weinstein GD: Photodynamic therapy with aminolevulinic acid topical solution and visible blue light in the treatment of multiple actinic keratoses of the face and scalp: investigator-blinded, phase 3, multicenter trials. Arch Dermatol 2004;140:41–46.
56 Pariser DM, Lowe NJ, Stewart DM, Jarratt MT, Lucky AW, Pariser RJ, Yamauchi PS: Photodynamic therapy with topical methyl aminolevulinate for actinic keratosis. results of a prospective randomized multicenter trial. J Am Acad Dermatol 2003;48:227–232.
57 Szeimies RM, Karrer S, Radakovic-Fijan S, Tanew A, Calzavara-Pinton PG, Zane C, Sidoroff A, Hempel M, Ulrich J, Proebstle T, Meffert H, Mulder M, Salomon D, Dittmar HC, Bauer JW, Kernland K, Braathen L: Photodynamic therapy using topical methyl 5-aminolevulinate compared with cryotherapy for actinic keratosis: a prospective, randomized study. J Am Acad Dermatol 2002;47:258–262.
58 Fritsch C, Homey B, Stahl W, Lehmann P, Ruzicka T, Sies H: Preferential relative porphyrin enrichment in solar keratoses upon topical application of delta-aminolevulinic acid methylester. Photochem Photobiol 1998;68:218–221.
59 Golub A, Gudgin Dickson EF, Kennedy JC, Marcus SL, Park Y, Pottier RH: The monitoring of ALA-induced protoporphyrin IX accumulation and clearance in patients with skin lesions by in vivo surface-detected fluorescence spectroscopy. Lasers Med Sci 1999;14:112–122.
60 Levulan Kerastick Important Information. http://www.dusapharma.com/levulan-product-information.html#fullpinfo.
61 Metvixia Cream (package insert). Oslo, ASA/Fort Worth, Galderma, 2008.
62 Szeimies R, Stockfleth E, Popp G, Borrosch F, Bruning H, Dominicus R, et al: Long-term follow-up of photodynamic therapy with a self-adhesive 5-aminolaevulinic acid patch: 12 months data. Br J Dermatol 2010;162:410–414.
63 Di Venosa G, Hermida L, Batlle A, et al: Characterisation of liposomes containing aminolevulinic acid and derived esters. J Photochem Photobiol B 2008;92:1–9.
64 Passos SK, de Souza PE, Soares PK, et al: Quantitative approach to skin field cancerization using a nanoencapsulated photodynamic therapy agent: a pilot study. Clin Cosmet Investig Dermatol 2013;6:51–59.
65 Dirschka T, Radny P, Dominicus R, Mensing H, et al: Photodynamic therapy with BF-200 ALA for the treatment of actinic keratosis: results of a multicentre, randomized, observer-blind phase III study in comparison with a registered methyl-5-aminolaevulinate cream and placebo. Br J Dermatol 2012;166:137–146.
66 Dirschka T, Radny P, Dominicus R, Mensing H, et al: Long-term (6 and 12 months) follow-up of two prospective, randomized, controlled phase III trials of photodynamic therapy with BF-200 ALA and methyl aminolaevulinate for the treatment of actinic keratosis. Br J Dermatol 2013;168:825–836.
67 Strasswimmer J, Grande DJ: Do pulsed laser produce an effective photodynamic therapy response? Lasers Surg Med 2006;38:22–25.
68 Wiegell S, Fabricius L, Stender I, Berne B, Kroon S, et al: A randomized, multicenter study of directed daylight exposure times of 1½ vs. 2½ h in daylight-mediated photodynamic therapy with methyl aminolaevulinate in patients with multiple thin actinic keratoses of the face and scalp. Br J Dermatol 2011; 164:1083–1090.
69 Gupta A, Paquet M: Network meta-analysis of the outcome ‘participant complete clearance’ in nonimmunosuppressed participants of eight interventions for actinic keratosis: a follow-up on a Cochrane review. Br J Dermatol 2013;169:250–259.
70 Vogler S, Tolley K: A network meta-analysis of the relative efficacy of treatments for actinic keratosis of the face or scalp in Europe. PLoS One 2014;9:e96829.
71 Tschen EH, Wong DS, Pariser DM, Dunlap FE, Houlihan A, Ferdon MB: Photodynamic therapy using aminolaevulinic acid for patients with nonhyperkeratotic actinic keratoses of the face and scalp: phase IV multicentre clinical trial with 12-month follow up. Br J Dermatol 2006;155:1262–1269.
72 Smith S, Piacquadio D, Morhenn V, Atkin D, Fitzpatrick R: Short incubation PDT versus 5-FU in treating actinic keratoses. J Drugs Dermatol 2003;2: 629–635.

73 Touma D, Yaar M, Whitehead S, Konnikov N, Gilchrest BA: A trial of short incubation, broad-area photodynamic therapy for facial actinic keratoses and diffuse photodamage. Arch Dermatol 2004;140:33–40.
74 Pariser D, McConnehey D, Bukhalo M, Matheson R, Guenthner S, et al: A phase II study of photodynamic therapy (PDT) with aminolevulinic acid HCl (ALA) 20% topical solution + blue light vs ALA topical solution vehicle + blue light using spot and broad area application and incubation times of 1, 2 and 3 hours for the treatment. J Am Acad Dermatol 2013; 68(suppl 1):AB156.
75 Apalla Z, Sotiriou E, Chovarda E, Lefaki I, Devliotou-Panagiotidou D, Ioannides D: Skin cancer: preventive photodynamic therapy in patients with face and scalp cancerization. A randomized placebo-controlled study. Br J Dermatol 2009;162:171–175.
76 Stasko T, Brown MD, Carucci J, et al: Guidelines for the management of squamous cell carcinoma in organ transplant recipients. Dermatol Surg 2004;30(4 pt 2):623.
77 Ulrich C, Bichel J, Euvrard S, et al: Topical immunomodulation under systemic immunosuppression: results of a multicentre, randomized, placebo-controlled safety and efficacy study of imiquimod 5% cream for the treatment of actinic keratoses in kidney, heart, and liver transplant patients. Br J Dermatol 2007;157S2:25–31.
78 Perrett CM, McGregor JM, Warwick J, et al: Treatment of posttransplant remalignant skin disease: a randomized intrapatient comparative study of 5-fluorouracil cream and topical photodynamic therapy. Br J Dermatol 2007;156:320–328.
79 De Graaf YG, Euvrard S, Bouwes Bavinck JN: Systemic and topical retinoids in the management of skin cancer in organ transplant recipients. Dermatol Surg 2004;30(4 pt 2):656–661.
80 Dragieva G, Hafner J, Dummer R, et al: Topical photodynamic therapy in the treatment of actinic keratoses and Bowen's disease in transplant recipients. Transplantation 2004;77:115–121.
81 Dragieva G, Prinz BM, Hafner J, et al: A randomized controlled clinical trial of topical photodynamic therapy with methyl aminolaevulinate in the treatment of actinic keratoses in transplant recipients. Br J Dermatol 2004;151:196–200.
82 De Graaf YGL, Kennedy C, Wolterbeek R, et al: Photodynamic therapy does not prevent cutaneous squamous-cell carcinoma in organ-transplant recipients: results of a randomized controlled trial. J Invest Dermatol 2006;126:569–574.
83 Wennberg AM, Stenquist B, Stockfleth E, Keohane S, Lear JT, Jemec G, Mork C, Christensen E, Kapp A, Solvsten H, Talme T, Berne B, Forschner T: Photodynamic therapy with methyl aminolevulinate for prevention of new skin lesions in transplant recipients: a randomized study. Transplantation 2008;86:423–429.
84 Willey A, Mehta S, Lee P: Reduction in the incidence of squamous cell carcinoma in solid organ transplant recipients treated with cyclic photodynamic therapy. Dermatol Surg 2010;36:652–658.
85 Kim R, Armstrong A: Nonmelanoma skin cancer. Dermatol Clin 2012;30:125–139.
86 Oseroff A, Shieh S, Frawley N, Cheney R, Blumenson L, et al: Treatment of diffuse basal cell carcinomas and basaloid follicular hamartomas in nevoid basal cell carcinoma syndrome by wide-area 5-aminolevulinic acid photodynamic therapy. Arch Dermatol 2005;141:60–67.
87 Athar M, Li C, Kim A, Spiegelman V, Bickers D: Sonic hedgehog signaling in basal cell nevus syndrome. Cancer Res 2014;74:4967–4975.
88 Sofen H, Peale F, Sharata H, Caro I, Gross K, Goldberg L, Hamilton T: Efficacy and safety of vismodegib in operable basal cell carcinoma: final results of a phase 2 trial. J Am Acad Dermatol 2014;70(suppl 1):AB135.
89 Clark C, Furniss M, Mackay-Wiggan J: Basal cell carcinoma: an evidence-based treatment update. Am J Clin Dermatol 2014;15:197–216.
90 Morton CA, Whitehurst C, McColl JH, Moore JV, MacKie RM: Photodynamic therapy for basal cell carcinoma – effect of tumour thickness and duration of photosensitiser application on response. Arch Dermatol 1998;134:248–249.
91 Morton C, Szeimies RM, Sidoroff A, Braathen L: European guidelines for topical photodynamic therapy. Part 1. Treatment delivery and current indications – actinic keratoses, Bowen's disease, basal cell carcionoma. J Eur Acad Dermatol Venereol 2013;27: 536–544.
92 Morton C, Szeimies R, Sidoroff A, Braathen L: European guidelines for topical photodynamic therapy. Part 2. Emerging indications – field cancerization, photorejuvenation and inflammatory/infective dermatoses. J Eur Acad Dermatol Venereol 2013;27: 672–679.
93 Basset-Seguin N, Bissonnette R, Girard C, et al: Concensus recommendations for the treatment of basal cell carcinomas in Gorlin syndrome with topical methylaminolaevulinate-photodynamic therapy. J Eur Acad Dermatol Venereol 2014;28:626–632.
94 Loncaster J, Swindell R, Slevin F, et al: Efficacy of photodynamic therapy as a treatment for Gorlin syndrome-related basal cell carcinomas. Clin Oncol (R Coll Radiol) 2009;21:502–508.
95 Pauwels C, Mazereeuw-Hautier J, Basset-Seguin N, et al: Topical methyl aminolevulinate photodynamic therapy for management of basal cell carcinomas in patients with basal cell nevus syndrome improves patient's satisfaction and reduces the need for surgical procedures. J Eur Acad Dermatol Venereol 2011; 25:861–864.

96 Chapas A, Gilchrest B: Broad area photodynamic therapy for treatment of multiple basal cell carcinomas in a patient with nevoid basal cell carcinoma syndrome. J Drugs Dermatol 2006;5(suppl 2):3–5.
97 Kabingu E, Oseroff A, Wilding G, Gollnick S: Enhanced systemic immune reactivity to a basal cell carcinoma associated antigen following photodynamic therapy. Clin Cancer Res 2009;15:4460–4466.
98 Basset-Seguin N, Ibbotson SH, Emtestam L, et al: Topical methylaminolaevulinate photodynamic therapy versus cryotherapy for superficial basal cell carcinoma: a 5 year randomized trial. Eur J Dermatol 2008;18:547–553.
99 Szeimies R, Ibbotson S, Murrell D, et al: A clinical study comparing methyl aminolevulinate photodynamic therapy and surgery in small superficial basal cell carcinoma (8–20 mm), with a 12-month follow-up. J Eur Acad Dermatol Venereol 2008;22:1302–1311.
100 Thissen M, Schroeter C, Neumann H: Photodynamic therapy with delta-aminolaevulinic acid for nodular basal cell carcinomas using a prior debulking technique. Br J Dermatol 2000;142:338–339.
101 Christensen E, Mork C, Skogvoll E: High and sustained efficacy after two sessions of topical 5-aminolaevulinic acid photodynamic therapy for basal cell carcinoma: a prospective and histological 10-year follow-up study. Br J Dermatol 2012;166:1342–1348.
102 Kuijpers DI, Thissen MR, Thissen CA, Neumann MH: Similar effectiveness of methyl aminolevulinate and 5-aminolevulinate in topical photodynamic therapy for nodular basal cell carcinoma. J Drugs Dermatol 2006;5:642–645.
103 Roozenboom M, Aardoom M, Nelemans P, Thissen M, Kelleners-Smeets N, Kuijpers D, Mosterd K: Fractionated 5-aminolevulinic acid photodynamic therapy after partial debulking versus surgical excision for nodular basal cell carcinoma: a randomized controlled trial with at least 5-year follow-up. J Am Acad Dermatol 2013;69:280–287.
104 Vinciullo C, Elliott T, Francis D, et al: Photodynamic therapy with topical methyl aminolaevulinate for difficult-to-treat basal cell carcinoma. Br J Dermatol 2005;152:765–772.
105 Rhodes LE, de Rie M, Enstrom Y, et al: Photodynamic therapy using topical methyl aminolevulinate vs surgery for nodular basal cell carcinoma: results of a multicenter randomized prospective trial. Arch Dermatol 2004;140:17–23.
106 Stender IM, Bech-Thomsen N, Poulsen T, Wulf HC: Photodynamic therapy with topical delta-aminolevulinic acid delays UV photocarcinogenesis in hairless mice. Photochem Photobiol 1997;66:493–496.
107 Hitz T, Ehler L, Hronung T, Voth H, Fortmeier I, et al: Preoperative characterization of basal cell carcinoma comparing tumour thickness measurement by optical coherence tomography, 20-MHz ultrasound and histopathology. Acta Derm Venereol 2012;92:132–137.
108 Morton CA, Horn M, Leman J, et al: A randomized, placebo-controlled, European study comparing MAL-PDT with cryotherapy and 5-fluorouracil in subjects with Bowen's disease. Arch Dermatol 2006;142:729–735.
109 Calzavara-Pinton P, Venturini M, Sala R: Methylaminolaevulinate-based photodynamic therapy of Bowen's disease and squamous cell carcinoma. Br J Dermatol 2008;159:137–144.
110 Lopez N, Meyer-Gonzalez T, Herrera-Acosta E, et al: Photodynamic therapy in the treatment of extensive Bowen's disease. J Dermatolog Treat 2012;23:428–430.
111 Markham T, Sheahan K, Collins P: Topical 5-aminolaevulinic acid photodynamic therapy for tumour-stage mycosis fungoides. Br J Dermatol 2001;144:1262–1263.
112 Quereux G, Brocard A, Saint-Jean M, et al: Photodynamic therapy with methyl-aminolevulinic acid for paucilesional mycosis fungoides: a prospective open study and review of the literature. J Am Acad Dermatol 2013;69:890–897.
113 Zane C, Venturini M, Sala R, Calzavara-Pinton P: Photodynamic therapy with methylaminolevulinate as a valuable treatment option for unilesional cutaneous T-cell lymphoma. Photodermatol Photoimmunol Photomed 2006;22:254–258.
114 Calzavara-Pinton PG, Rossi MT, Sala R; Italian Group for Photodynamic Therapy: A retrospective analysis of real-life practice of off-label photodynamic therapy using methyl aminolevulinate (MAL-PDT) in 20 Italian dermatology departments. Part 2. Oncologic and infectious indications. Photochem Photobiol Sci 2013;12:158–165.
115 Nestor MS, Gold MH, Kauvar AN, Taub AF, Geronemus RG, Ritvo EC, Goldman MP, Gilbert DJ, Richey DF, Alster TS, Anderson RR, Bank DE, Carruthers A, Carruthers J, Goldberg DJ, Hanke CW, Lowe NJ, Pariser DM, Rigel DS, Robins P, Spencer JM, Zelickson BD: The use of photodynamic therapy in dermatology: results of a consensus conference. J Drugs Dermatol 2006;5:140–154.

George Martin, MD
Dr. George Martin Dermatology Associates
41 East Lipoa Street, Suite 21
Kihei, Maui, HI 96753 (USA)
E-Mail drmauiderm@gmail.com

Gold MH (ed): Cosmetic Photodynamic Therapy. Aesthet Dermatol. Basel, Karger, 2016, vol 3, pp 123–132
DOI: 10.1159/000439343

How I Use Photodynamic Therapy with 5-Aminolevulinic Acid in My Clinical Practice

Dore J. Gilbert

Newport Dermatology and Laser Associates, Newport Beach, Calif., USA

Abstract

Since the early 1990s, the use of photodynamic therapy (PDT) with 5-aminolevulinic acid (ALA) has become a primary or adjunctive therapy for a variety of skin conditions. Advantages include its selectivity for abnormal tissue, efficacy over large anatomical fields, manageable side effects, and excellent cosmetic outcomes. Although FDA cleared only for the treatment of nonhypertrophic actinic keratosis (AK) of the face and scalp using a blue light source, PDT with ALA photosensitizing agent has been used off-label to treat acne, nonmelanoma skin cancers, photodamage, sebaceous skin, and other skin disorders. Pre- and posttreatment procedures are well documented, and light sources are readily available. Cosmetic benefits encourage patients to request other cosmetic treatments, thus improving practice revenue. This chapter provides an updated guide to implementing ALA-PDT into clinical practice.

Introduction

The use of photodynamic therapy (PDT) has expanded considerably during the past decade because the technique is effective against a variety of dermatologic conditions [1]. Advantages of PDT are its proven ability to enhance both clinical and cosmetic outcomes [2, 3]. Although FDA cleared only for the treatment of nonhypertrophic actinic keratosis (AK) of the face and scalp using the blue light source (BluU®; DUSA Pharmaceuticals, Inc. Wilmington, Mass., USA), PDT with 5-aminolevulinic acid (ALA) photosensitizing agent (as Levulan® Kerastick®; DUSA Pharmaceuticals) has been used off label to treat acne, nonmelanoma skin cancers, photodamage, sebaceous skin, and other skin conditions [4]. The other well-known photosensitizing agent, methyl aminolevulinate (MAL; Metvixia®; Galderma Laboratories, Fort Worth, Tex.,

Table 1. Consensus recommendations for light sources, number of treatments, and treatment intervals for ALA-PDT

Dermatologic condition	Light source, preferred/ alternate/other	Treatments, n (interval)	Comment
AKs, superficial BCC	Blue/PDL[a], IPL[b]/ green, yellow, red	1–2 (3–5 or 2 weeks)[c]	
Photodamage/ cosmetic enhancement	IPL[b] (blue for skin type VI)/blue, PDL[a]/ green, yellow[d]	At least 2 (2–4 or 1 weeks)[c] depending on severity of damage	Typically 5 treatments at 2- to 3-week intervals; 3 treatments include ALA
Acne	PDL→blue (5 min)/ blue (8 min)/green, red, IPL, yellow	1–3 (2–3 weeks)[e]	Treat flares immediately; 6- to 12-month clearance typical
Sebaceous skin, rosacea, rhinophyma	PDL[f], blue/IPL[b]/ green[f], yellow, red	1–2 (3–5 or 2 weeks)[c]	

PDL = Pulsed dye laser. *Preferred* sources produce the most significant response for the lesion type and may cause response without ALA (i.e. IPL for photodamage or PDL for acne). *Alternate* sources result in substantial effectiveness against the lesion type. *Other* sources have unproven effectiveness against the lesion type (i.e. 532-nm light for acne). Adapted from Nestor et al. [4], with permission. [a] Fluences that avoid bruising. [b] Standard photorejuvenation settings by patient type. [c] Increase ALA incubation time if necessary in second and subsequent treatments. [d] Optimum is IPL, PDL, or green (532 nm) followed by blue light for 5 min. (The author of this paper recommends 10 min of blue light treatment.) [e] For skin types IV–VI, ALA incubated 30 min for first treatment. [f] Double or triple pulsing on lesion recommended.

USA), is FDA cleared for use in combination with a red light source (Aktilite; Galderma Laboratories) for the treatment of nonhypertrophic AK of the face and scalp. MAL is also approved in Europe for the treatment of basal cell carcinoma (BCC) for which conventional therapy is unsuitable [5]. To the author's knowledge, MAL is not yet available in the United States.

ALA-PDT has attracted dermatologists' attention because the topically administered ALA accumulates more quickly in abnormal tissue than in normal tissue, conferring selectivity for the target tissue. ALA enters the epidermis and is converted to protoporphyrin IX (PpIX), which, in the presence of oxygen and light energy of the appropriate wavelength, is converted to singlet oxygen, a metastable intermediate that selectively destroys the target tissue [4].

A variety of laser or light sources can activate ALA-induced PpIX (table 1) [3, 4]. Therefore, physicians whose practice includes laser- or light-based treatments may already have the equipment to implement ALA-PDT. The author uses blue light

(BluU) for many applications because it provides light at 417 nm, the maximum absorption peak of PpIX. Since ALA diffusion is limited to the epidermis [6] and sebaceous glands [7], healing occurs quickly and with minimal risks of infection and scarring [6, 8].

Clinical Practice

Since experience with MAL is limited in the United States [5], the author of this chapter focuses on PDT with ALA. Guidelines for implementing ALA-PDT have been published [9] and are updated in this chapter. The author continues to use ALA-PDT for the treatment of AK, nonmelanoma skin cancer, acne, sebaceous hyperplasia, and photodamage of facial and nonfacial areas. New uses of PDT (alone or in combination with other modalities) in the author's practice include treatment of actinic cheilitis, chemoprevention of AK and nonmelanoma skin cancers in organ transplant patients, and prevention of multiple recurrent malignant lesions in large anatomical fields. An advantage of PDT is that it permits cyclical treatment of large lesional areas in one to two sessions with an excellent cosmetic outcome [10–12]. In organ transplant patients with multiple recurrent malignant lesions, the author uses imiquimod or ALA-PDT for chemoprevention. This decision is supported by Sotiriou et al. [13] who showed that MAL-PDT and imiquimod 5% (used individually) prevented the development of new AK lesions in patients with changes in field cancerization. In immunocompetent patients, the author treats individual recurrent lesions of squamous cell carcinoma or BCC with surgery unless multiple lesions are present. Patients for whom ALA-PDT is contraindicated are treated with liquid nitrogen, imiquimod, or 5-fluorouracil (5-FU).

Applications

Actinic Keratoses

The author uses ALA-PDT as both a first-line and adjunctive option for the treatment of AKs. Topical therapies such as 5-FU may require up to 4 weeks of treatment during which posttreatment erythema persists, whereas with ALA-PDT, erythema subsides within 1 week unless multiple treatments are required. Treatment sessions may be scheduled so that erythema does not affect patient lifestyles. The author treats the scalp, chest, arms, hands, and legs, especially in patients with actinic porokeratosis.

The author has successfully combined 5-FU and single-session ALA-PDT in sequence for the treatment of AK [14]. In this study, 15 patients with multiple and diffuse facial AK lesions underwent a 6-day course of treatment in which they applied 5-FU each night for 5 days and received ALA-PDT on the 6th day. On the day of PDT, ALA covered the entire face for 30–45 min under low-intensity visible light. ALA was removed and faces were treated with one pass of intense pulsed light (IPL). One month later, 90% of AK lesions had resolved in 14 of the 15 patients and erythema had cleared 7–10 days after ALA-PDT. AK resolution persisted for at least 1 year. The combined modality had produced redness and scaling that persisted for only 7–10 days, whereas with 5-FU alone the redness may last for 4 weeks.

Acne and Sebaceous Skin

ALA-PDT has been shown in numerous studies to be useful in the treatment of acne [4]. Many acne patients prefer to avoid extended use of antibiotics and seek an alternative to isotretinoin because of the latter's adverse effects and regulations that limit its use. Patients with acne-induced erythematous scars notice that their skin often returns to a normal color after ALA-PDT. The use of ALA-PDT to treat other sebaceous disorders has been described [4].

Actinic Cheilitis

The author uses an ALA-PDT procedure similar to that of Sotiriou et al. [15], who recently described a sequential use of MAL-PDT with imiquimod 5% for the treatment of actinic cheilitis. Its prompt treatment is important because this condition may progress to squamous cell carcinoma with a relatively high risk of metastasis [15].

New Applications

A variety of difficult-to-treat cutaneous disorders such as molluscum contagiosum, hidradenitis suppurativa, cutaneous leishmaniasis, cutaneous T-cell lymphoma, extramammary Paget's disease, Hailey-Hailey disease, keratosis pilaris, keratoacanthoma, perioral dermatitis, mycosis fungoides, nevus sebaceous, psoriasis, localized scleroderma, and warts have been treated with ALA-PDT [4].

Clinical and Financial Benefits

Cosmetic Effects

ALA-PDT improves cosmetic appearance when used alone or in combination with other modalities [3]. Improvement is comparable to that obtained with a 30% trichloroacetic acid peel, but healing is quicker, and scarring and other serious adverse effects occur less often [8]. In the author's practice, ALA-PDT-induced cosmetic improvement includes noticeably reduced hyperpigmentation, erythema, photodamage, fine lines, and pore size.

Enhanced Light Effects

The use of IPL for activation in PDT reduces the number of IPL treatments required for photorejuvenation and improves the patient's overall cosmetic appearance in the author's practice. Turnover of pigmented cells increases and telangiectasias are reduced, thus decreasing erythema as well.

Financial Effects

The author charges USD 300–1,000 per PDT treatment session, depending on the light source and the amount of ALA needed for the procedure. Patients consider ALA-PDT more efficient and less expensive than traditional topical therapies for a variety of skin conditions. This preference may be because PDT can be performed in 1 day with reduced inflammation and recovery time compared to 5-FU, imiquimod, or diclofenac sodium [16]. ALA-PDT has increased practice revenue, especially when used to improve cosmesis. The cosmetic benefit often results in inquiries about cosmetic procedures such as dermal filler injections, botulinum toxin injections, PhotofacialP, leg vein removal, and cosmetic surgery.

Light source prices range from USD 8,000 for a blue light to USD 100,000 for an IPL system. Continuous and pulsed light-emitting diodes (LEDs) for red and blue light are priced at approximately USD 30,000. High-quality digital imaging equipment for patient photographs costs USD 4,000–6,000 or higher. A single Levulan Kerastick costs USD 300.00 and a single treatment session requires 1 or 2 Kerasticks. (One Kerastick is paid for by Medicare.) Other consumables depend on the light source, and their costs are negligible, especially for blue light.

Insurance coverage for ALA-PDT is limited to FDA-cleared indications, such as AK. Use of Levulan or BluU to treat off-label conditions such as acne, photodamage, sebaceous hyperplasia, and rosacea is usually not covered. To increase the chance for coverage, the physician should ask the insurance company directly to precertify a specific patient.

Reimbursement differs among insurance companies and among regions of the United States.

The Current Procedural Terminology codes for Levulan Kerastick in PDT are CPT 99201 and 99211 for new and established patients, respectively. The Healthcare Common Procedure Coding System drug code for Levulan Kerastick is HCPCS J7308. Activating Levulan is coded by 96567 for PDT with the BluU and the 17000 destruction codes for laser treatment (17000 for the initial lesion, 17003 for lesions 2–14, and 17004 for lesions 15 and beyond). To the author's knowledge, there are no specific criteria that patients must meet before the insurance company will cover the treatment of AK with ALA-PDT, nor do patients need to fail other treatments to obtain this coverage.

Implementation

ALA-PDT is easy to learn and perform, especially when the light source is already in the office and used for other procedures. If a new light source is introduced, the physician can train staff as soon as he or she becomes comfortable in its operation. Physicians without PDT experience should be as consistent as possible with the light activation technique and ALA incubation times (30–60 min). AK is simple to treat whereas acne is difficult because many patients are of school age, absence from school may become an issue, and many treatment sessions may be required.

Spatial requirements are limited to the space needed by the light source. The BluU requires only 2 square feet and stands in the corner of a room, whereas LED units can be positioned on a desk. Most light sources need 110 V, so special wiring is not needed.

Levulan Kerastick

The composition and terminology of the Levulan Kerastick are quoted below from the package insert (DUSA Pharmaceuticals, Inc.) [17].

LEVULAN® KERASTICK® (aminolevulinic acid HCl) for Topical Solution, 20%, a porphyrin precursor, contains the hydrochloride salt of aminolevulinic acid (ALA), an endogenous 5-carbon aminoketone… The LEVULAN KERASTICK for Topical Solution applicator is a two component system consisting of a plastic tube containing two sealed glass ampules and an applicator tip. One ampule contains 1.5 ml of solution vehicle comprising alcohol USP (ethanol content = 48% v/v), water, laureth-4, isopropyl alcohol, and polyethylene glycol. The other ampule contains 354 mg of ALA HCl as a dry solid. The applicator tube is enclosed in a protective cardboard sleeve and cap. The 20% topical solution is prepared just prior to the time of use by breaking the ampules and mixing the contents by shaking the LEVULAN KERASTICK applicator. The term 'ALA HCl' refers to unformulated active ingredient, 'LEVULAN KERASTICK for Topical Solution' refers to the drug product in its unmixed state, 'LEVULAN KERASTICK Topical Solution' refers to the mixed drug product (in the applicator tube or after application), and 'LEVULAN KERASTICK' refers to the applicator only.

Patients and Scheduling

Patients suitable for ALA-PDT have sufficient disposable income and will tolerate the downtime for cosmetic treatments. Typical patient characteristics include photodamaged skin, red or brown discoloration, and diffuse AKs. Patients whose acne was not improved by oral and topical medications are also appropriate for ALA-PDT.

Avoidance of sun exposure after a PDT session is critical to a positive outcome. For this reason, PDT sessions are scheduled during the late afternoon. Patients desiring to return to their jobs as soon as possible are treated on Thursdays or Fridays so they can recover from posttreatment erythema and scaling during the weekend, and go to work on Monday. Women can apply makeup and men often resume shaving by the 5th day after treatment.

The Initial Consultation

The physician, a registered nurse, or both begin by explaining the efficacy and safety of ALA-PDT to patients. A nurse may explain ALA-PDT to candidates for Photofacial treatments while the physician discusses ALA-PDT as an option for acne or AK. Patients are also shown photographs of patients before and after ALA-PDT.

1 Photograph the patient with both digital and Polaroid cameras. Place photographs on the patient's chart.

2 Instruct patient to continue topical or systemic medications.

3 Treat the target area with a 5-FU (Fluoroplex, 1% topical cream, Aqua Pharmaceuticals, West Chester, Pa., USA) for 5 days [11].

4 Wash the target area with soap and water or alcohol.

5 Perform either single-pass microdermabrasion, acetone scrub, or both to remove the keratin layer and increase ALA penetration. In teenaged patients, scrub to the patient's comfort level.

6 Gently crush ALA ampules with the fingers and shake the Kerastick for approximately 3 min, keeping the sponge end up.

7 Apply ALA liberally to the skin, using extra pressure to the target lesions. Spread the solution uniformly with gloved fingertips. Avoid mucous membranes.

8 Allow ALA to incubate for at least 30–60 min.

9 Remove ALA with soap and water only if using large amounts of gel during IPL treatment. Otherwise, leave ALA on the skin.

10 Wash the patient's face after treatment is completed.

Fig. 1. ALA-PDT pretreatment protocol (adapted from Gilbert [9], with permission).

As with any procedure, patients are informed in advance about possible adverse effects which are typically mild and transient. They are shown photos of mild and severe reactions to ALA-PDT. Posttreatment instructions are explained in detail, and patients are encouraged to contact the physician, physician assistant, or registered nurse with questions.

Preparing for Treatment

The author's pretreatment protocol for all skin conditions is shown in figure 1. The patient is photographed and the target area is treated with 5-FU for 5 days. The previous protocol [9] did not include the latter step. On the day of the procedure, the target area is washed and the keratin layer removed to improve ALA penetration. ALA is applied uniformly and allowed to incubate 30–60 min before irradiation with light.

Treatment Protocol

In patients undergoing ALA-PDT for the first time, ALA incubation is approximately 1 h for most skin conditions. ALA incubation may be extended to 2–3 h or overnight in patients (1) whose response to previous ALA-PDT treatments showed minimal erythema or limited cosmetic improvement or (2) being treated for severe AK, superficial BCC, or squamous cell carcinoma. Responses to earlier treatments are used to guide treatment parameters for subsequent sessions. For example, if a patient's most recent session resulted in minimal erythema, the physician increases the ALA incubation time or the fluence in the next session.

Table 2. Duration of irradiation with LED systems in ALA-PDT for acne, photodamage, AK, and other applications

LED device		Duration, min
Omnilux	Alderm, Irvine, Calif., USA	
Red		15
Blue		12
GentleWaves	Light BioScience LLC,	14
Red	Virginia Beach, Va., USA	
Yellow		15

Reproduced from Gilbert [9].

To treat AK, the author currently incubates ALA for 1 h and activates ALA-induced PpIX by IPL (Lumenis® One; Lumenis Inc., San Jose, Calif., USA) using a 560-nm filter, 16 J/cm^2 fluence, and 4.0-ms double pulsing with a 20-ms delay. IPL-exposed areas are further irradiated with blue light for 2–10 min (unless patient discomfort is excessive) with cooling by a patient-operated hand fan. Alternatively, the author may lengthen pulse durations to increase IPL contact time with the skin.

As shown in table 2, ALA-PDT with LED irradiation for 12–15 min is effective against acne, AK, photodamage, and other applications.

Evaluating Results

For patients with AK, responses to ALA-PDT are evaluated 1 week, 1 month, and 1 year after treatment. Improvement is usually evident at 1 month. Acne patients are treated once monthly for 4 months and again as needed. Improvement is noticeable after the second or fourth treatment. Patients with sebaceous hyperplasia are treated once and evaluated at 1 month.

Adverse effects after ALA-PDT have been minimal and transient in the author's practice. Anesthesia is usually not necessary. However, patients must be educated and urged to minimize sun exposure for 2 weeks after ALA-PDT to avoid phototoxic reactions.

Physicians should also consider the risks of bacterial infection, persistent erythema, exacerbation of herpetic infections, postinflammatory hyperpigmentation, hypopigmentation, and hypertrophic scars after ALA-PDT. The author manages bacterial infections with antibiotic medications and cleansing. Erythema is treated with topical steroids, and hyperpigmentation is treated with hydroquinone. Patients with a history of herpetic infection receive a prophylactic antiviral agent (Valtrex 1 g b.i.d.) the day before, the day of, and the day after ALA-PDT. Rare hypertrophic scars are treated with intralesional steroids. (The author has never observed hypertrophic scars due to ALA-PDT.)

Other adverse effects and their treatment have been presented [8] and are summarized in order of decreasing frequency: erythema (hydrocortisone ointment), flakiness (moisturizer), edema (ice pack), crusting (water and vinegar soaks), oozing/vesiculation (vinegar soaks), pain (OTC analgesic), hyperpigmentation (none), and blistering (ice pack).

Posttreatment Care

Recovery time after ALA-PDT is less than that of CO_2 and Er:YAG laser therapy.

Epidermal reepithelialization occurs quickly because ALA-PDT causes minimal damage to the dermis [6]. Redness, scaling, and slight swelling are common during the initial 12 h. Swelling (most pronounced around the eyes) persists and redness may increase during the next 24 h. Ice packs reduce swelling and discomfort. Skin reactivity increases with long ALA incubation time [8].

On the day of ALA-PDT, patients apply ice packs to the treated areas, take pain medication as needed, and avoid sun exposure for the first 24–48 h to allow residual ALA-induced PpIX to clear the skin [4]. Exposure of residual PpIX to ultraviolet (UV) radiation activates PpIX and causes itching, burning, and other manifestations of phototoxicity [6]. Hydrocortisone may be applied and patients may take a shower. Between days 2 and 7, patients should continue pain medications and ice packs, treat blisters and edematous areas as needed, and protect treated areas from sun exposure. Blisters have been reported in patients receiving ALA-PDT with red light [18]. Blisters, if they develop, may be soaked in diluted white vinegar followed by ice packs, drying, and petrolatum or hydrocortisone (1%) application every 4–6 h during waking hours. When scaling and redness are no longer apparent (4–5 days after treatment), healing is complete. Female patients may apply makeup (preceded by moisturizer). Most patients comply with these instructions [8]. Patients should shield the treated areas from sunlight for 2 weeks after treatment because the new epidermal cells are sensitive to UV radiation. Sun block (at least 30 SPF) may be used during this period. Titanium dioxide-zinc oxide may be used to block UVA and UVB light [4]. If the treated area is red after crusting has stopped, patients may apply green-based cover-up to conceal redness.

The author's experience shows that the severity of ALA-PDT wounds increases with fluence, ALA incubation time, and the number of passes. Wound severity also varies with the activation wavelength and light source [8].

ALA-PDT is a nonsurgical treatment for a variety of skin disorders. It is safe, effective, and easy to perform. Patients consider ALA-PDT more efficient and less expensive than traditional topical therapies. Pre- and posttreatment procedures are well documented, and light sources are readily available. Cosmetic benefits encourage patients to request other cosmetic treatments, thus improving practice revenue. For these reasons, the author continues to use ALA-PDT and will expand its use as new applications become available.

The author plans to combine microneedling (Dermapen™) with ALA-PDT to enhance ALA penetration for the treatment of AK and Bowen's disease in organ transplant patients.

References

1 Gold MH: Therapeutic and aesthetic uses of photodynamic therapy. Part one of a five-part series. The use of photodynamic therapy in the treatment of actinic keratoses and in photorejuvenation. J Clin Aesthet Dermatol 2008;1:32–37.

2 Taub AF: Photodynamic therapy in dermatology: history and horizons. J Drugs Dermatol 2004; 3(suppl):8S–25S.

3 Gold MH, Goldman MP: 5-Aminolevulinic acid photodynamic therapy: where we have been and where we are going. Dermatol Surg 2004;30:1077–1083.

4 Nestor MS, Gold MH, Kauvar AN, Taub AF, Geronemus RG, Ritvo EC, Goldman MP, Gilbert DJ, Richey DF, Alster TS, Anderson RR, Bank DE, Carruthers A, Carruthers J, Goldberg DJ, Hanke CW, Lowe NJ, Pariser DM, Rigel DS, Robins P, Spencer JM, Zelickson BD: The use of photodynamic therapy in dermatology: results of a consensus conference. J Drugs Dermatol 2006;5:140–154.

5 Gold MH: Therapeutic and aesthetic uses of photodynamic therapy. Part five of a five-part series. ALA-PDT and MAL-PDT what makes them different. J Clin Aesthet Dermatol 2009;2:44–47.

6 Kennedy J, Pottier R: Endogenous protoporphyrin IX, a clinically useful photosensitizer for photodynamic therapy. J Photochem Photobiol B 1992;14: 275–292.

7 Hongcharu W, Taylor CR, Chang Y, Aghassi D, Suthamjariya K, Anderson RR: Topical ALA-photodynamic therapy for the treatment of acne vulgaris. J Invest Dermatol 2000;115:183–192.

8 Gilbert DJ: Post-Treatment Care for Photodynamic Therapy with Topical 5-Aminolevulinic Acid. US Dermatology. London, Touch Briefings, 2006, pp 85–87.

9 Gilbert DJ: Incorporating photodynamic therapy into a medical and cosmetic dermatology practice. Dermatol Clin 2007;25:111–118.

10 Dragieva G, Hafner J, Dummer R, Schmid-Grendelmeier P, Roos M, Prinz BM, Burg G, Binswanger U, Kempf W: Topical photodynamic therapy in the treatment of actinic keratoses and Bowen's disease in transplant recipients. Transplantation 2004;77:115–121.

11 O'Reilly Zwald F, Brown M: Skin cancer in solid organ transplant recipients: advances in therapy and management. Part II. Management of skin cancer in solid organ transplant recipients. J Am Acad Dermatol 2011;65:263–279.

12 Willey A, Mehta S, Lee PK: Reduction in the incidence of squamous cell carcinoma in solid organ transplant recipients treated with cyclic photodynamic therapy. Dermatol Surg 2010;36:652–658.

13 Sotiriou E, Apalla Z, Vrani F, Lallas A, Chovarda E, Ioannides D: Photodynamic therapy vs. imiquimod 5% cream as skin cancer preventive strategies in patients with field changes: a randomized intraindividual comparison study. J Eur Acad Dermatol Venereol 2015;29:325–329.

14 Gilbert DJ: Treatment of actinic keratoses with sequential combination of 5-fluorouracil and photodynamic therapy. J Drugs Dermatol 2005;4:161–163.

15 Sotiriou E, Lallas A, Goussi C, Apalla Z, Trigoni A, Chovarda E, Ioannides D: Sequential use of photodynamic therapy and imiquimod 5% cream for the treatment of actinic cheilitis: a 12-month follow-up study. Br J Dermatol 2011;165:888–892.

16 Braathen LR, Morton CA, Basset-Seguin N, Bissonnette R, Gerritsen MJ, Gilaberte Y, Calzavara-Pinton P, Sidoroff A, Wulf HC, Szeimies RM: Photodynamic therapy for skin field cancerization: an international consensus. International Society for Photodynamic Therapy in Dermatology. J Eur Acad Dermatol Venereol 2012;26:1063–1066.

17 Levulan® Kerastick® Important Information. http://www.dusapharma.com/levulan-product-information.html#fullpinfo (accessed August 16, 2014).

18 Fijan S, Honigsmann H, Ortel B: Photodynamic therapy of epithelial skin tumours using delta-aminolaevulinic acid and desferrioxamine. Br J Dermatol 1995;133:282–288.

Dore J. Gilbert, MD, Medical Director
Newport Dermatology and Laser Associates
1441 Avacado, Suite 806
Newport Beach, CA 92660 (USA)
E-Mail lazrdoc@pacbell.net

Author Index

Clementoni, M.T. 64

Foley, P. 36

Gilbert, D.J. 123
Gold, M.H. VII, 1
Goldman, M.P. 8

Martin, G. 103

Munavalli, G.S. 64

Peterson, J.D. 8

Roscher, M.B. 64

Schieber, A.C. 85

Taub, A.F. 85

Subject Index

Acne vulgaris
  photodynamic therapy
    clinical protocols 96–98
    complications 98, 99
    dosage 92, 93
    incubation time 90
    light sources
      blue light 87, 88
      intense pulsed light 89, 90
      pulsed dye laser 89
      red light 89
    mechanism of action 86, 87
    outcomes 90, 91
    overview 126
    photosensitizers 93–96
    prospects 99, 100
  treatment overview 85, 86
Actinic cheilitis, 5-aminolevulinic acid photodynamic therapy 126
Actinic keratosis (AK)
  5-aminolevulinic acid photodynamic therapy
    advantages 11, 12, 126, 127
    clinical technique
      chart 20
      incubation time 19, 129, 130
      irradiation 130
      light source selection 19, 21, 124
      posttreatment considerations 21, 22, 131
      preoperative considerations 19
      skin preparation 18
    combination therapy 18
    consultation 128, 129
    disadvantages 12
    exclusion criteria 30
    organ transplant recipient considerations 22, 23
    outcomes by light source
      blue light 12, 13, 16
      intense pulsed light 17, 130, 131
      red light 17
      yellow-orange light with pulsed dye laser 16, 17
    overview 125, 126
    pretreatment protocol 129
    published trials 13–15
    side effects and complication management 30, 31
  chemoprevention photodynamic therapy 106–110
  epidemiology 38
  methyl aminolevulinate photodynamic therapy
    5-aminolevulinic acid photodynamic therapy-controlled studies 51
    cryotherapy-controlled studies 50, 51
    daylight photodynamic therapy 53, 55
    inclusion criteria 40
    mechanism of action 38, 39
    meta-analysis of studies 39–45, 50, 52, 53
    outcome measures and outcomes 40, 46–50
    overview 38
    placebo-controlled studies 50
    regimen comparison study 52
  natural history 37, 38
  treatment overview 11
Aging skin, *see* Photorejuvenation
AK, *see* Actinic keratosis
ALA, *see* 5-Aminolevulinic acid

5-Aminolevulinic acid (ALA)
acne vulgaris photodynamic therapy, *see* Acne vulgaris
actinic keratosis photodynamic therapy, *see* Actinic keratosis
chemoprevention, *see* Chemoprevention
history of use 4–6, 9, 64, 123
indications 125, 126
Levulan Kerastick composition and terminology 128
light sources for photodynamic therapy 124, 125
pharmacology 10
photorejuvenation, *see* Photorejuvenation

Basal cell carcinoma, *see* Chemoprevention
Blue light
acne vulgaris photodynamic therapy 87, 88
5-aminolevulinic acid photodynamic therapy for actinic keratosis 12, 13, 16
photorejuvenation 24
sebaceous gland hyperplasia photodynamic therapy 87, 88

Cancer chemoprevention, *see* Chemoprevention
Chemoprevention
actinic keratosis 106–110
skin cancer
basal cell carcinoma 114–116
cutaneous T-cell lymphoma 117, 118
epidemiology 103, 104
nonmelanoma skin cancer 110–114
overview of approaches 104
photodynamic therapy 104, 105
squamous cell carcinoma 116, 117
Cutaneous T-cell lymphoma, *see* Chemoprevention

Daylight photodynamic therapy, actinic keratosis 53, 55

Economics, photodynamic therapy 127

Hematoporphyrin, history of use 2, 3
Hematoporphyrin purified derivative (HPD), history of use 3, 4
HPD, *see* Hematoporphyrin purified derivative

IAA, *see* Indole-2-acetic acid
ICG, *see* Indocyanine green
Indocyanine green (ICG), acne vulgaris photodynamic therapy 95
Indole-2-acetic acid (IAA), acne vulgaris photodynamic therapy 96
Intense pulsed light (IPL)
acne vulgaris photodynamic therapy 89, 90
5-aminolevulinic acid photodynamic therapy
actinic keratosis 17
photorejuvenation 28, 29, 65–67, 73
advantages 126
photorejuvenation 28, 29, 65–67, 73
sebaceous gland hyperplasia photodynamic therapy 89, 90
IPL, *see* Intense pulsed light

Levulan Kerastick, *see* 5-Aminolevulinic acid

MAL, *see* Methyl aminolevulinate
Methyl aminolevulinate (MAL)
acne vulgaris photodynamic therapy 94, 95
actinic keratosis photodynamic therapy, *see* Actinic keratosis
chemoprevention, *see* Chemoprevention
history of use 5, 6, 9, 123, 124
photorejuvenation, *see* Photorejuvenation
Methylene blue, acne vulgaris photodynamic therapy 95, 96

Organ transplant recipient
actinic keratosis
chemoprevention photodynamic therapy considerations 105, 110–114
photodynamic therapy considerations 22, 23

PDT, *see* Photodynamic therapy
Photodynamic therapy (PDT), *see also specific indications*
economics 127
historical perspective 1–6, 64
lasers and light sources 10, 11
mechanism of action 9
Photorejuvenation
5-aminolevulinic acid photodynamic therapy
clinical technique 30, 69–78
combination therapy 29
exclusion criteria 30
indications 73
outcomes by light source

blue light 24
intense pulsed light 28, 29, 65–67, 73
red light 24, 28, 73
yellow-orange light with pulsed dye laser 29
photodynamic effect enhancement 67–69
postoperative care 72
published clinical studies 25–27
roller device 72, 74
side effects and complication management 30, 31
methyl aminolevulinate photodynamic therapy 56–60
photodamaged skin
overview 23, 24, 37, 65
treatment options 65
PpIX, *see* Protoporphyrin IX
Protoporphyrin IX (PpIX)
chemoprevention photodynamic therapy 106
history of use 4, 5, 8
Pulsed dye laser
acne vulgaris photodynamic therapy 89
5-aminolevulinic acid photodynamic therapy for actinic keratosis 16, 17
photorejuvenation 29
sebaceous gland hyperplasia photodynamic therapy 89

Red light
acne vulgaris photodynamic therapy 89
5-aminolevulinic acid photodynamic therapy for actinic keratosis 17
photorejuvenation 24, 28, 73
sebaceous gland hyperplasia photodynamic therapy 89
Rejuvenation, *see* Photorejuvenation

Sebaceous gland hyperplasia
photodynamic therapy
complications 98, 99
dosage 92, 93
incubation time 90
light sources
blue light 87, 88
intense pulsed light 89, 90
pulsed dye laser 89
red light 89
mechanism of action 86, 87
outcomes 90, 91
photosensitizers 93–96
prospects 99, 100
treatment overview 86
Skin cancer chemoprevention, *see* Chemoprevention
Skin rejuvenation, *see* Photorejuvenation
Squamous cell carcinoma, *see* Chemoprevention

T-cell lymphoma, *see* Chemoprevention